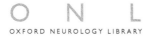

O N L
OXFORD NEUROLOGY LIBRARY

Vertigo and
Dizziness

Date: 1/19/18

616.841 BUK
Büki, Béla,
Vertigo and dizziness /

D1600846

O N L

OXFORD NEUROLOGY LIBRARY

Vertigo and Dizziness

Béla Büki MD PhD

Dept. of Otolaryngology
County Hospital Krems
Krems an der Donau, Austria

Alexander A. Tarnutzer MD

Dept. of Neurology
University Hospital Zurich
Zurich, Switzerland

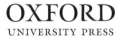

OXFORD
UNIVERSITY PRESS

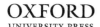

OXFORD
UNIVERSITY PRESS

Great Clarendon Street, Oxford, OX2 6DP,
United Kingdom

Oxford University Press is a department of the University of Oxford.
It furthers the University's objective of excellence in research, scholarship,
and education by publishing worldwide. Oxford is a registered trade mark of
Oxford University Press in the UK and in certain other countries

Published in the United States of America by Oxford University Press
198 Madison Avenue, New York, NY 10016, United States of America

British Library Cataloguing in Publication Data
Data available

Library of Congress Control Number: 2013938570

ISBN 978–0–19–968062–7

Printed in Great Britain
by Ashford Colour Press Ltd, Gosport, Hampshire

Contents

Foreword

There can be few physicians so dedicated to their art that they do not experience a slight decline in spirits on learning that their patient's complaint is of giddiness. This frequently means that after exhaustive enquiry it will still not be entirely clear what it is that the patient feels wrong and even less so why he feels it.

> Matthews W.B. (1963) *Practical Neurology. Oxford, Blackwell.*

A pithy quip from Bryan Matthews (1920–2001), Professor of Clinical Neurology at Oxford (1970–1987), and one of the finest clinical neurologists of his day. But even then he was not quite right in his assessment of the dismal state of neuro-otology fifty years ago. Queen Square—where Drs Hallpike, Dix, Cawthorne, and Carmichael were busily making important contributions to our understanding of the vestibular system—was not so far from Oxford. But as only one of the awesome foursome, Dr Carmichael, was a neurologist (Hallpike and Cawthorne (Sir Terence) were otologists, and (Margaret) Dix was neither), Matthews probably had not heard of them; or if he had, he did not take much notice. But from that acorn, what a mighty oak has grown! With some understanding of basic vestibular physiology, it is now possible, in my view, to make a reasonable diagnosis on history and examination in about 80% of dizzy patients at the first consultation, with only an audiogram and a video head impulse test to help; and to be able to treat successfully about 80% of them (the Pareto Principle at work). This little book distils the practical aspects of these advances, so that any practitioner with an interest in treating dizzy patients can acquire state-of-the art knowledge and have a chance of approximating this hit rate.

Prof Gábor Michael Halmágyi
February 2013, Sydney, Australia

Acknowledgements

The authors would especially like to thank Dominik Straumann from the Department of Neurology, University Hospital Zurich, Zurich, Switzerland for his useful comments during his meticulous and motivated work reviewing and correcting all chapters.

They also thank Jonathan A. Edlow from the Department of Emergency Medicine, Beth Israel Deaconess Medical Center and Harvard Medical School, Boston for having reviewed Chapter 2 (Dizziness as emergency).

Note to the Reader

The authors report no conflict of interest. The manuscript has been completed solely on the basis of available scientific evidence, without any commercial considerations.

Abbreviations

4-AP	4-aminopyridine
ABR	auditory brainstem repsonses
ACD	alcoholic cerebellar degeneration
AED	anti-epileptic drugs
AICA	anterior inferior cerebellar artery
AVM	arteriovenous malformation
AVS	acute vestibular syndrome
Isolated AVS	defined by Tarnutzer *et al* (2011) as 'isolated acute vestibular syndrome (with or without hearing loss) as occurring in the absence of focal neurologic signs such as hemiparesis, hemisensory loss, gaze palsy' lasting more than 24 hours.
AP	action potential (in electrocochleography)
BA	basilar artery
BPPV	benign paroxysmal positional vertigo
BPVC	benign paroxysmal vertigo of childhood
BVD	bilateral vestibular deafferentation
CANVAS	cerebellar ataxia, neuropathy, vestibular areflexia syndrome
ChT	chemotherapy
CIDP	chronic inflammatory demyelinating polyneuropathy
CJD	Creutzfeldt-Jakob disease
sCJD	sporadic Creutzfeldt-Jakob disease
CNS	central nervous system
COX	cyclooxygenase
CPV	central positional vertigo
CRP	C-reactive protein
CSD	chronic subjective dizziness
CSF	cerebrospinal fluid
CT	computed tomography
CCT	cranial computed tomography
CVI	chronic vestibular insufficiency
DRPLA	dentatorubral-pallidoluysian atrophy
DVA	dynamic visual acuity
DWI	diffusion-weighted imaging

EA	episodic ataxia
Ecochg	electrocochleography
ECG	electrocardiogram
ED	emergency department
EEG	electroencephalogram
EGFR	epidermal growth factor receptor
ENMG	electroneuromyography
FLAIR	fluid-attenuated inversion recovery
FRDA	Friedreich's ataxia
FXTAS	fragile-X tremor ataxia syndrome
GABA	gamma-aminobutyric acid
GAD	glutamic acid decarboxylase
HER	human epidermal growth factor receptor
HINTS	Head Impulse test, searching for direction-changing Nystagmus and Test of Skew deviation
HIT	head impulse test
hHIT	horizontal head impulse test
vHIT	video head impulse test
HSMN IV	hereditary sensory and autonomic neuropathy
IHS	international headache society
INFARCT	Impulse Normal or Fast-phase Alternating or Refixation on Cover Test
ISHL	idiopathic sudden hearing loss
LA	left anterior
LARP	left anterior, right posterior (defining the SCCs oriented in a specific plane)
LP	left posterior
LVAS	large vestibular aqueduct syndrome
MD	Menière's disease
MRA	magnetic resonance angiography
MRI	magnetic resonance imaging
MS	multiple sclerosis
MSA	multiple system atrophy
MSA-C	multiple system atrophy of cerebellar type
NF1	neurofibromatosis type 1; Recklinghausen's disease
NF2	neurofibromatosis type 2
NPH	normal pressure hydrocephalus
Oc90	otoconin 90

OTR	ocular tilt reaction
PAN	periodic alternating nystagmus
PCD	paraneoplastic cerebellar degeneration
PD	Parkinson's disease
PICA	posterior inferior cerebellar artery
PLF	perilymph fistula
PNP	peripheral polyneuropathy
POTS	postural orthostatic tachycardia syndrome
PSP	progressive supranuclear palsy
RA	right anterior
RALP	right anterior, left posterior (defining the SCCs oriented in a specific plane)
RBD	REM-sleep behavioural disorders
REM	rapid eye movement
RP	right posterior
RTK	receptor tyrosine kinase
RVAS	rotational vertebral artery syndrome
SAOA	sporadic adult-onset ataxia of unknown origin
SCA	superior cerebellar artery
SCAs	spinocerebellar ataxias
SCA1	spinocerebellar ataxia type 1
SCA2	spinocerebellar ataxia type 2
SCA3	spinocerebellar ataxia type 3
SCA6	spinocerebellar ataxia type 6
SCA7	spinocerebellar ataxia type 7
SCA8	spinocerebellar ataxia type 8
SCA10	spinocerebellar ataxia type 10
SCA12	spinocerebellar ataxia type 12
SCA17	spinocerebellar ataxia type 17
SCC	semicircular canal
SCCD	semicircular canal dehiscence
SP	summating potential (in electrocochleaography)
SPS	stiff person syndrome
SREAT	steroid-responsive encephalopathy associated with autoimmune thyroiditis
SSCDS	superior semicircular canal dehiscence syndrome
TIA	transient ischemic attack

TLOC	transient loss of consciousness
UPDRS	unified Parkinson's disease rating scale
uVD	unilateral vestibular deafferentation
VA	vertebral artery
VAD	vertebral artery dissection
VEGF	vascular endothelial growth factor
VEGFR1	VEGF receptor 1
VEMP	vestibular evoked myogenic potential
oVEMP	ocular VEMP (when testing the vestibulo-ocular reflex)
cVEMP	cervical VEMP (when testing the vestibulo-collic reflex)
VM	vestibular migraine
VN	vestibular neuritis
VOR	vestibulo-ocular reflex
VP	vestibular paroxysmia
VS	schwannoma of the vestibular nerve
WE	Wernicke's encephalopathy

Chapter 1

Introduction

Key points

- Major advances in both pathophysiology and treatment strategies have made neurotology a fast developing field.
- Recent insights and revolutionary diagnostic methods have helped to define novel dizziness entities and design effective therapeutic methods.
- There are new, practical bedside tests for differentiating between peripheral and possibly life-threatening central causes of vertigo and dizziness—applicable even in the general practice.
- Short, repetitive vestibular stimuli applied using the principle of evoked potentials allow high-resolution examination of vestibular end organs in cases with 'vertigo of attrition'.
- Neurologists should be aware of otological facts, and otologists should think about the central nervous system (CNS) when examining and treating vertigo and dizziness.

1.1 Silent revolution

In the last two to three decades, a silent revolution has occurred in neurotology. A growing understanding of physiologic principles has led to new examination techniques, and modern diagnostics have helped to define new entities of vestibular pathology. This, in turn, has resulted in a decrease in the number of clinical cases for which no diagnosis could be made. Also, advanced, effective therapeutic strategies have been established. Today, the latest innovative examination methods make it possible to assess vestibular function with an unprecedentedly high resolution: individual semicircular canals (SCCs) or otolithic organs can be tested separately in a fast, reliable, and clinically meaningful way. These new developments have by no means moved neurotology away from frontline medicine into an ivory tower; never has it been possible to know more about potential diagnoses in cases with acute vertigo at the bedside than today.

1.2 Milestones on a dizzy road

This evolution could not have happened without revolutionary discoveries. In 1988, the head impulse test (HIT) was described (Halmagyi and Curthoys 1988); by now its significance in differentiating between cerebellar stroke and peripheral neuritis has been clearly established (Tarnutzer *et al* 2011). In 1992, Epley demonstrated that, in benign paroxysmal positional vertigo (BPPV), otoconia are not necessarily glued to the cupula as previously presumed but instead move freely in the posterior canal and can be flushed out by a special sequence of movements (equivalent to a backward somersault in two phases). This method gave doctors the potential for miraculous healings. In 1992, Colebatch and Halmagyi applied revolutionary new methods for vestibular stimulation based on the principle of evoked responses and described the short latency reaction of cervical muscles to loud clicks originating in the saccule. This opened the floodgates; due to the ensuing torrential stream of publications, vestibular evoked potentials have become a standard test, making selective utricular and saccular functional measurements possible. With quantitative video-based head impulse testing now available (Weber *et al* 2008), the function of individual SCCs can be assessed reliably in an everyday clinical setting, providing, together with vestibular evoked potentials, a powerful tool to assess all parts of the peripheral vestibular organs individually.

The quest for the 'Holy Grail' of neurotology, for the ultimate, causative therapy of Menière's disease (MD), goes on. However, it has been possible to register a partial success—at least to effectively alleviate symptoms without cutting the vestibular nerve. Although spontaneously improving in many cases, MD may cause severe complaints, making normal everyday life almost impossible. After having been suggested in the 1950s (Schuknecht 1957), vestibular ablation using aminoglycosides fell into disfavour because of the high rate of sensorineural hearing loss accompanying it. The topic received a boost in 2000, when Carey *et al* showed that even a single intratympanic injection of gentamicin caused a reduction in SCC function (with a latency of several weeks) similar to that of repeated injections. It did not cause complete inhibition of the angular vestibulo-ocular reflex (VOR), as is the case with surgical deafferentation, but the relatively mild effect was obviously sufficient to obtain a symptom-free period of at least several months. Single, infrequent injections with gentamicin apparently do not harm hearing. Since then, after having been successfully tested against placebo in randomized studies, low dose intratympanic gentamicin has become the 'state of the art' therapy for MD.

Thanks to otoconia research, three-dimensional labyrinth reconstructions, and three-dimensional vector-nystagmography, a conclusive picture about otoconial debris movement in BPPV has recently emerged. It is also easier to understand its variants, such as BPPV without nystagmus or the (not so rare) peripheral downbeat nystagmus in the Dix-Hallpike position (Cambi *et al* 2013).

Even in the relatively recent past, new entities have been discovered. In 1998, Minor *et al* described the SCC dehiscence syndrome, which explains several bizarre complaints such as pressure-induced vertigo or when patients say 'Doctor, I hear the movements of my eyes!' Since then, the principle has been generalized into the concept of a mobile 'third window' on the labyrinth and allowed otologists to understand cases with pseudoconductive hearing loss, when ear operations cannot improve hearing. The advent of high-resolution vestibulometry has made it possible to define a new entity that may explain a clinically mysterious, obviously peripheral syndrome with vertigo, vomiting (sometimes even with hearing loss), but without spontaneous nystagmus: isolated inferior vestibular neuritis (VN; Halmagyi *et al* 2002). Future observations will reveal how frequent this syndrome is. However, it is not too early to say that its appearance will lower the number of cases with 'vertigo of unknown origin'.

1.3 Otology, neurology, and the general practice

These and other major discoveries have made neurotology a fast developing, fascinating field arising between neurology and otology. The examiner has two important aims when diagnosing and treating patients with vertigo or dizziness. First, to identify and treat potentially dangerous causes of acute dizziness or vertigo (this should be done even in the general practice or in the emergency unit); second, to find the cause and bring relief in cases of 'vertigo of attrition', those cases in which recurrent vertigo attacks make normal life impossible. In this book, we would like to help the reader to achieve both aims by reviewing classical knowledge and new developments in diagnostics and effective therapies, presenting the essential principles of neurotology in an accessible way.

References and Further Reading

Carey J. P., Minor L. B., Peng G. C. Y. *et al.* (2000) Changes in the three-dimensional angular vestibulo-ocular reflex following intratympanic gentamicin for Ménière's disease. *JARO.* **3**, 430–43.

Cambi J., Astore S., Mandalà M. *et al.* (2013) Natural course of positional down-beating nystagmus of peripheral origin. *J Neurol.* [Epub ahead of print].

Colebatch J. G. and Halmagyi G. M. (1992) Vestibular evoked potentials in human neck muscles before and after unilateral vestibular deafferentation. *Neurology.* **42**, 1635–6.

Epley J. M. (1992) The canalith repositioning procedure: for treatment of benign paroxysmal positional vertigo. *Otolaryngol Head Neck Surg.* **107**, 399–404.

Halmagyi G. M., Aw S. T., Karlberg M. *et al.* (2002) Inferior vestibular neuritis. *Ann N Y Acad Sci.* **956**, 306–13.

Halmagyi G. M. and Curthoys I. S. (1988) A clinical sign of canal paresis. *Arch Neurol.* **45**, 737–9.

Minor L. B., Solomon D., Zinreich J. S. *et al.* (1998) Sound- and/or pressure-induced vertigo due to bone dehiscence of the superior semicircular canal. *Arch Otolaryngol Head Neck Surg.* **124**, 249–58.

Schuknecht H. F. (1957) Ablation therapy in the management of Meniere's disease. *Acta Otolaryngol (Stockh).* **132**, 1–42.

Tarnutzer A. A., Berkowitz A. L., Robinson K. A. *et al.* (2011) Does my dizzy patient have a stroke? A systematic review of bedside diagnosis in acute vestibular syndrome. *CMAJ.* **183**, E571–92.

Weber K. P., Aw S. T., Todd M. J. *et al.* (2008) Head impulse test in unilateral vestibular loss: vestibulo-ocular reflex and catch-up saccades. *Neurology.* **70**, 454–63.

4

Dizziness as emergency

5

2.1 Introduction

The most important task for the clinician in the emergency department (ED) is to identify potentially serious, life-threatening causes. Dizziness (including vertigo, presyncope, disequilibrium, and other unspecified dizziness) as the chief symptom accounts for roughly 3–6% of all ED admissions (Newman-Toker et al 2008b; Kroenke and Mangelsdorff 1998). Even among younger patients, 10% of cases have a more serious underlying cause (Newman-Toker et al 2008b). Based on an analysis of the diagnoses made in US emergency departments, Newman-Toker et al (2008b) concluded that dizziness is not attributed to a vestibular disorder in most ED cases. The most frequent **benign causes** of dizziness were vasovagal syncope (6.6% of all visits) followed by VN (5.6%), migraine (1.1%), benign paroxysmal position vertigo (BPPV; 0.7%), and orthostatic hypotension (0.6%). Ménière's disease (MD) had a frequency of 0.3%. Among the more dangerous causes presenting with dizziness, fluid electrolyte disorders were the most common (5.6%), followed by cardiac arrhythmias (3.2%), transient ischaemic attack (TIA; 1.7%), anaemia (1.6%), hypoglycaemia (1.4%), angina (0.9%), myocardial infarction (0.8%), and stroke/intracerebral haemorrhage (0.5%).

Disorders presenting with dizziness as the leading symptom may be broadly classified into two main categories: transient dizziness and dizziness lasting for more than a day. Transient complaints lasting for seconds, minutes, or hours have been traditionally attributed to more benign, peripheral vestibular dysfunction such as BPPV or MD. However, TIAs or primary cardiovascular disorders, which when left untreated can be potentially serious, can also cause transient dizziness. Apparently, it is not possible to classify entities into 'serious' or 'benign' according to the character of complaints—vertigo or imbalance—either. First, patients do not accurately specify their complaints (patients often change the 'category' of acute dizziness within ten minutes if asked a second time, and they often endorse two categories simultaneously (Newman-Toker et al 2007)); second, even if patients do accurately specify the character of their complaints, both categories may include cases with serious diagnoses. Cerebellar or brainstem stroke can present with either imbalance or vertigo. It has been suggested recently that even cardiovascular pathologies may cause **vertigo** more frequently than previously thought. In a meta-analysis in a group of cardiovascular patients who experienced dizziness, 63% had vertigo in addition to other symptoms, and 37% had vertigo alone (Newman-Toker et al 2008a).

Potentially dangerous entities (such as posterior circulation stroke) often cause dizziness for longer than 24 hours and fulfil the criteria for AVS, in which vertigo is accompanied by nausea, vomiting, unsteady gait, and nystagmus. In this group, the self-limiting, benign peripheral entity vestibular neuritis (VN) is more frequent than the potentially life-threatening cerebellar stroke. In the last few years, new, simple bedside tests have been suggested that have high sensitivity and specificity in differentiating between the two, even in the first few hours when the neuroradiologic diagnosis may not be accurate or available (Tarnutzer et al 2011).

Central vestibular dysfunction (mostly due to stroke) may often be misdiagnosed and falsely contributed to a benign, peripheral cause. Although computed tomography (CT) has poor sensitivity in posterior fossa acute stroke, and even diffusion-weighted magnetic resonance imaging (MRI) misses possibly one in five posterior fossa strokes when carried out early (Tarnutzer et al 2011), follow-up radiological evaluations are carried out relatively infrequently after discharge from the ED (Edlow et al 2008). If a posterior fossa stroke has been missed, diagnoses are often corrected during the stay of the patients or in the light of the results of follow-up examinations (Royl et al 2011). Exact evaluation is important; patients discharged home from the ED with complaints of dizziness or vertigo will have subsequent vascular events more frequently (4.7%) than those without dizziness/vertigo (1.8%) (Lee et al 2012).

2.2 Acute dizziness for longer than a day with focal neurologic signs

Focal neurologic symptoms, when present in a dizzy patient, indicate a potentially dangerous central cause; however, their absence does not make a purely peripheral cause more probable (Tarnutzer et al 2011). Although dizziness (Anagnostou et al 2010) may occur in hemispheric stroke with special localizations (e.g. temporal lobe), the most important entity with dizziness as leading symptom for longer than a day is posterior circulation stroke. Branches of the main cerebellar arteries also supply the brainstem; accordingly, occlusion of more proximal branches may cause accompanying brainstem signs and cranial nerve dysfunction. Some of these are, however, in most cases easy to miss (such as loss of pain and temperature sensation, hoarseness, diplopia, or Horner syndrome) and have to be specifically searched for. Variations of arterial supply and anastomoses are common; therefore, clinical presentation of posterior circulation stroke may be variable. Although rare, basilar migraine should be a valid differential diagnostic entity in cases with dizziness, headache, and brainstem symptoms.

2.3 AVS: dizziness for more than 24 hours without neurologic signs

Approximately 25 ± 15% of all AVS cases are probably caused by stroke, with about 50% of these cases lacking focal neurological signs (Tarnutzer et al 2011). These latter cases may be difficult to separate from entities such as VN, the most frequent cause of peripheral-type AVS. This hypothetically viral, benign, and self-limiting entity is more frequent than its central counterpart, the 'vestibular pseudoneuritis' caused by cerebellar or brainstem stroke. Differentiating between the two is important, since cerebellar stroke can be fatal without close monitoring. Ten to twenty per cent of patients—perhaps after having been discharged from the ED with a misdiagnosis of peripheral-type AVS, e.g. due to acute VN—deteriorate during the days following cerebellar stroke due to brainstem compression and hydrocephalus, with the swelling peaking on the third day after infarction (Edlow et al 2008).

In their systematic review, Tarnutzer et al (2011) defined 'isolated acute vestibular syndrome (with or without hearing loss) as occurring in the absence of focal neurologic signs such as hemiparesis, hemisensory loss, gaze palsy' and lasting more than 24 hours. About 10–20% of patients who visited the ED with acute dizziness had AVS. The most common peripheral cause was VN. The most common central causes were posterior fossa ischaemic stroke (79% of all central causes), haemorrhage (4%), and multiple sclerosis (MS; 11%). These central causes may mimic VN.

2.3.1 Differentiating between VN and posterior circulation stroke

VN invariably causes dysfunction of the vestibulo-ocular reflex (VOR) and asymmetry of the firing rate in the brainstem vestibular nuclei. This asymmetry leads to spontaneous nystagmus which does not change its direction according to gaze (the fast component always beating away from the affected ear). Due to the dysfunctional VOR, the patient cannot fixate a stationary target during passive, small amplitude, high velocity head rotations towards the involved side (horizontal head impulse test (hHIT)). Instead of holding the gaze, the eyes turn with the head and the gaze, driven by a retinal error signal, catches up afterwards with a compensatory saccade to the healthy side. Since the VOR is intact in cases with infarction in the territory of the posterior inferior and superior cerebellar arteries, hHIT constitutes an easy and fast method to differentiate between the two. When the hHIT is pathological towards the direction of the slow phase of the spontaneous nystagmus in AVS, a peripheral cause on this side may be suspected. With some practice, this test may be carried out even without specialization in neurotology. The presence of spontaneous nystagmus does not hinder the evaluation, because the test is highly pathological in acute cases, the compensatory saccade being easily noticeable. If, in contrast, the hHIT is bidirectionally normal, this result must raise the possibility of stroke. A positive hHIT alone, however, may lure the examiner into a false sense of safety, such as, for example, in cases with infarctions of the anterior inferior cerebellar artery (AICA), because these may involve the inner ear or the vestibular nuclei, causing combined, central, and peripheral vestibular dysfunction. In these cases, the hHIT may be positive despite the presence of a potentially dangerous cerebellar stroke, falsely indicating a benign peripheral lesion. Therefore, the examiner should search for other central ocular motor signs. Since AICA-infarcts usually cause central eye–movement disturbances, e.g. due to lesions of the neuronal circuits responsible for gaze holding and vertical ocular alignment, the search for subtle ocular motor signs (direction-changing nystagmus and skew deviation) and their combination with the hHIT should increase sensitivity. Therefore, Kattah et al (2009) suggested the application of a three-step bedside test consisting of the **H**ead **I**mpulse test, searching for direction-changing **N**ystagmus, and **T**est of **S**kew deviation (HINTS). The authors proposed a second acronym for the composite HINTS test results predicting stroke: **I**mpulse **N**ormal or **F**ast-phase **A**lternating or **R**efixation on **C**over **T**est (INFARCT). A meta-analysis showed that the composite HINTS examination had a sensitivity of 100% and a specificity of 96% for stroke, giving better results than diffusion-weighted MRI in ruling out stroke in early (i.e. within 24 to 48 hours) presentations of AVS (Tarnutzer et al 2011). The 96% specificity means that, although rare, false positive cases may nevertheless occur. Sometimes VN may cause primary position 'peripheral' skew deviation (reported in 4% of patients with peripheral AVS compared to 25% with central-type AVS (Kattah et al 2009)). In such cases, spontaneous nystagmus, positive hHIT, and skew deviation might suggest infarction of the AICA-territory; thus the HINTS may be false positive. However, in acute VN, ipsilateral acute hearing loss is usually missing, while admission and observation combined with repeated radiological evaluation (MRI) may clarify diagnosis.

Whereas a single transient prodromal episode of dizziness within a few days before the occurrence of an AVS is probably nonspecific (being reported with high frequency both for VN and stroke), multiple transient prodromal episodes of dizziness over weeks to months favour stroke (Tarnutzer et al 2011). Other red flags for stroke possibly include sudden and severe craniocervical pain (frequently reported in cerebellar stroke and vertebral artery dissection but less so in VN) and recent trauma (increasing the risk for vertebrobasilar dissection, although absence of trauma is insufficient to exclude dissection).

2.3.2 Limitations of diagnostic tests, misdiagnoses

Analysis of nystagmus and eye movements, the head impulse test (HIT), and searching for subtle neurologic signs such as sensory disturbances, cranial nerve dysfunction, limb-ataxia, and gait are important components of the bedside examination of acutely dizzy patients. Negative hHIT in spite of spontaneous nystagmus, direction-changing nystagmus on eccentric gaze, purely vertical or torsional spontaneous nystagmus, and/ or focal neurological signs should alert the examiner and suggest a possibly serious underlying cause. In cases when patients cannot walk or stand unaided, stroke might be suspected. There are, however, vestibular examinations which should not be part of the initial examination battery of an acutely dizzy patient. Head motion exacerbates symptoms and signs in AVS. Because of the strong intolerance of head motion, positional testing (such as the Dix-Hallpike test) is not indicated in the acute stage of prolonged vertigo with spontaneous nystagmus.

CT has low sensitivity in verifying acute ischaemic cerebellar stroke, possibly because ischaemic lesions in the posterior fossa are particularly difficult to demonstrate among the artefacts created by the surrounding bone. In a recent study of Hwang et al (2012), the sensitivity of non-contrast cerebral CT carried out in the first 30 hours was 42%. Examiners should be aware of this limitation.

Caloric irrigation may also have its limitations in AVS, since it may give reduced responses even in posterior inferior cerebellar artery (PICA)-territory infarctions (Newman-Toker et al 2008c); this limits its potential as a tool for localizing the site of the lesion. Savitz et al (2007) reviewed misdiagnosed cases of cerebellar infarctions. The initial diagnoses in this group of 15 relatively young patients included migraine, toxic encephalopathy, gastritis, meningitis, myocardial infarction, and polyneuropathy. The overall mortality was high (40%), and half of the survivors had disabling deficits. Most frequent causes of misdiagnoses were failure to recognize focal neurologic symptoms (pathologic gait, eye-movement disturbances, and disorders of limb strength and coordination) and overreliance on negative CT scans of the brain.

2.4 Transient dizziness

By definition, AVS lasts longer than 24 hours. Dizziness spells, which are shorter and self-limiting, are classified as transient. In spite of the self-limiting complaints, it is important to establish a diagnosis in these cases as well, since they may have potentially dangerous causes, and at the time of admission the vertigo/dizziness is a 'developing story'—it is not clear how long it will last. In this group, we find several peripheral vestibular entities for which the HINTS battery may indicate central disturbance while the attack is still going on. This persuades the clinician to stay on the safe side and search for central pathologies. To err in this direction is not as dangerous as having false negative results with respect to stroke.

2.4.1 Cardiac arrhythmia and TIA

As mentioned, cardiovascular disease may cause dizziness and even vertigo, representing 21% of all ED consultations with a main complaint of acute dizziness (Newman-Toker et al 2008b). Besides fluid and electrolyte disorders (5.6%), cardiac arrhythmia (3.2%) and TIA of the posterior circulation (1.7%) are the most frequently observed potentially dangerous causes of transient dizziness in the ED setting. TIAs are defined as complaints lasting less than 24 hours; in 2002, a new definition was proposed by the TIA Working Group that includes 'clinical symptoms typically lasting less than one hour' (Albers et al 2002). Transient vertebrobasilar insufficiency is associated with short-lasting visual symptoms (e.g. diplopia and visual field defects), sudden falls with or without transient loss of consciousness, dysarthria, and perioral numbness, but surprisingly often presents with isolated vertigo only. In a study by Grad and Baloh (1989), 62% of patients with vertebrobasilar insufficiency reported at least one episode of isolated vertigo; in 19% of the cases, vertigo was the initial symptom. Newer data suggests that stroke occurs rather soon after the first TIA complaints; vertigo or dizziness attacks occurring longer than 3–6 months are rarely caused by vertebrobasilar insufficiency but may be related to slowly progressive vasculopathy (Tarnutzer *et al* 2011). This stresses the importance of early diagnosis (including search for causative factors such as cardioembolism) and treatment to prevent stroke.

2.4.2 BPPV

Among peripheral vestibular entities causing transient vertigo and dizziness, BPPV is the most frequent in the general population. In the ED, cases with acute VN seem to be more prevalent, probably because of the more severe complaints presented (Newman-Toker *et al* 2009). Although BPPV may cause chronic recurrent vertigo lasting for seconds over weeks and months, its first bout may manifest itself (usually in the morning, when getting up from the bed) as a true vestibular emergency for several hours. However, even in acute BPPV, vertigo and positional nystagmus subside when the patient is lying completely motionless. In cases, when otolithic debris moves to and fro in the **horizontal semicircular canals**, sometimes 'lying-down nystagmus' may develop (see Chapter 5). This consists of a transient, purely horizontal nystagmus, which occurs when, during the examination, the patient reclines from sitting into a supine position, and debris moves to the most inferior part of the horizontal canal. This nystagmus may be misinterpreted as spontaneous nystagmus.

In BPPV, hHIT carried out as a bedside test is typically bilaterally negative, and usually there is no accompanying acute hearing loss. VN occurring in the superior branch of the nerve predisposes to BPPV; therefore a pathologic hHIT in combination with provocation manoeuvres indicating BPPV instead relates to a chronic unilateral vestibular deficit and suggests previous superior branch VN with sequential posterior canal BPPV.

2.4.3 MD

The duration of an attack with MD should not exceed approximately two hours—at least, the strongest vertigo should subside within that time; unspecific post-attack discomfort and slight post-attack nystagmus may last longer. Depending on the individual time course, MD may present with a complete, transient vestibular loss (with spontaneous nystagmus, positive hHIT away from the fast phase) or with a vestibular irritation. In the latter case, spontaneous vestibular firing increases on the involved side, causing an excitatory spontaneous nystagmus with a fast phase towards the involved side with a bilaterally normal hHIT. After a longer attack, a transient 'post-attack' spontaneous nystagmus may occur in the excitatory direction, again with a normal hHIT to both sides. Even if the symptoms later subside, the results of the HINTS examination battery raise the possibility of a central pathology (such as posterior circulation TIA).

2.4.4 Neuritis of the inferior branch of the vestibular nerve

This entity has not been known until relatively recently, and since it seems not to be frequent, its features have not been evaluated. Still, we mention it here because its peculiar pattern may confound the HINTS examination battery. The inferior vestibular nerve innervates the posterior semicircular canal (SCC) and the saccule. Isolated vestibular dysfunction sometimes affects only this nerve branch, causing transient dizziness (for hours), nausea, and, interestingly, frequently also hearing loss. There is a diagonal vestibular asymmetry between the involved posterior SCC on one side and the anterior one on the other side. Patients might have no spontaneous nystagmus at all, or if any, it might be slight, downbeating, and torsional. On hHIT, lateral canal function should be normal, but posterior canal function should be impaired on one side (as assessed by the diagonal HIT). The inferior vestibular nerve also innervates the saccule and, using new methods of vestibular evoked potential testing, it is possible to demonstrate saccular hypofunction.

2.4.5 Vestibular migraine (VM)–vertebral artery dissection (VAD)

Headache is a common complaint in strokes in the posterior circulation: nearly 10% of patients with cerebellar infarction have headache (Edlow et al 2008). In these cases, migraine is often a misdiagnosis (Savitz et al 2007). Tarnutzer et al (2011) found in their systematic review that, although VM is seldom considered as a cause of AVS, relatively young patients with VAD often received the misdiagnosis of migraine. It is almost a cliché that VM is the chameleon among disorders causing dizziness. It leads to variable symptoms, making differential diagnosis difficult. Its duration may last from several hours to three days; presenting complaints may include central oculomotor signs, gait ataxia, dysarthria, and impaired hearing. However, in migraine, the worst dizziness is usually an aura phenomenon and, as such, subsides after one hour; headache associated with VM is often relatively mild and may be adequately managed with aspirin, non-steroid anti-inflammatory drugs, or other mild analgesics. Other aura phenomena, such as scintillating scotoma, may also serve as a useful sign for the diagnosis.

2.5 Conclusions

The cause of acute dizziness in the ED is frequently benign. However, some patients have serious, even potentially life-threatening conditions. Evaluation of dizzy patients should rely on carefully noting relevant details concerning its history (e.g. head or neck trauma, cardiovascular risk factors). It is important to note accompanying complaints such as (occipital) headache, hearing loss or increased tinnitus, fever, and chest pain. The duration or recurrence of the symptoms is a significant detail. Complaints with a duration longer than 24 hours help to exclude transient dizziness syndromes. Careful physical examination is indispensable, including searching for spontaneous nystagmus, subtle oculomotor signs, or cranial nerve dysfunction. Ability to sit or stand unaided and limb coordination should be examined. Close clinical monitoring is crucial. Patients with suspected cerebellar or brainstem stroke should be managed in a stroke centre with a neurological intensive care unit. In more benign peripheral vestibular diseases, symptoms may be alleviated by supportive measures and vestibular sedatives.

References and Further Reading

Albers G. W., Caplan L. R., Easton J. D. et al. (2002) Transient ischemic attack—proposal for a new definition. N Engl J Med. **347**, 1713–16.

Anagnostou E., Spengos K., Vassilopoulou S. et al. (2010) Incidence of rotational vertigo in supratentorial stroke: a prospective analysis of 112 consecutive patients. J Neurol Sci. **290**, 33–6.

Edlow J. A., Newman-Toker D. E., Savitz S. I. (2008) Diagnosis and initial management of cerebellar infarction. *Lancet Neurol.* **7**, 951–64.

Grad A. and Baloh R. W. (1989) Vertigo of vascular origin. Clinical and electronystagmographic features in 84 cases. *Arch Neurol.* **46**, 281-4.

Halmagyi G. M., Aw S. T., Karlberg M. *et al.* (2002) Inferior vestibular neuritis. *Ann N Y Acad Sci.* **956**, 306–13.

Hwang D.Y., Silva G.S., Furie K.L., *et al.* (2012) Comparative sensitivity of computed tomography vs. magnetic resonance imaging for detecting acute posterior fossa infarct. *J Emerg Med.* **42**, 559–65.

Kattah J. C., Talkad A. V., Wang D. Z. *et al.* (2009) HINTS to diagnose stroke in the acute vestibular syndrome: three-step bedside oculomotor examination more sensitive than early MRI diffusion-weighted imaging. *Stroke.* **40**, 3504–10.

Kroenke K. and Mangelsdorff A. D. (1989) Common symptoms in ambulatory care: incidence, evaluation, therapy, and outcome. *Am J Med.* **86**, 262–6.

Lee C. C., Ho H. C., Su Y. C. *et al.* (2012) Increased risk of vascular events in emergency room patients discharged home with diagnosis of dizziness or vertigo: a 3-year follow-up study. *PLoS One.* **7**, e35923.

Newman-Toker D. E., Camargo C. A. Jr, Hsieh Y. H. *et al.* (2009) Disconnect between charted vestibular diagnoses and emergency department management decisions: a cross-sectional analysis from a nationally representative sample. *Acad Emerg Med.* **16**, 970–7.

Newman-Toker D. E., Cannon L. M., Stofferahn M. E. *et al.* (2007) Imprecision in patient reports of dizziness symptom quality: a cross-sectional study conducted in an acute care setting. *Mayo Clin Proc.* **82**, 1329–40.

Newman-Toker D. E., Dy F. J., Stanton V. A. *et al.* (2008a) How often is dizziness from primary cardiovascular disease true vertigo? A systematic review. *J Gen Intern Med.* **23**, 2087–94.

Newman-Toker D. E., Hsieh Y. H., Camargo C. A. Jr *et al.* (2008b) Spectrum of dizziness visits to US emergency departments: cross-sectional analysis from a nationally representative sample. *Mayo Clin Proc.* **83**, 765–75.

Newman-Toker D. E., Kattah J. C., Alvernia J. E. *et al.* (2008c) Normal head impulse test differentiates acute cerebellar strokes from vestibular neuritis. *Neurology.* **70**, 2378–85.

Royl G., Ploner C. J., Leithner C. (2011) Dizziness in the emer-gency room: diagnoses and misdiagnoses. *Eur Neurol.* **66**, 256–63.

Savitz S. I., Caplan L. R., Edlow J. A. (2007) Pitfalls in the diagnosis of cerebellar infarction. *Acad Emerg Med.* **14**, 63–8.

Tarnutzer A. A., Berkowitz A. L., Robinson K. A. *et al.* (2011) Does my dizzy patient have a stroke? A systematic review of bedside diagnosis in acute vestibular syndrome. *CMAJ.* **183**, E571–92.

Vestibular physiology

3.1 **Hair cells**

Vestibular hair cells measure accelerations of the head by transforming inertial movements of SCC fluid or otoconia into neural signals through deflection of stereocilia. Deflection towards the higher stereocilia increases the rate of neurotransmitter release at the basal part of the cell. Deflection in the other direction decreases transmitter emission (Figure 3.1). In SCCs, the hair cells and ampullae are positioned in such a way that **excitation** of hair cells occurs by acceleration of the head towards the ipsilateral side. In birds and mammals, two types of hair cells have been described: type I and type II. Type I hair cells are globular and are completely surrounded by a large calyx nerve terminal. Type II hair cells are cylindrical and contact several small synaptic terminals. The difference between the two classes may be clinically significant: gentamicin, a vestibulotoxic antibiotic, causes greater loss of type I than type II hair cells.

3.2 **Vestibulo-ocular reflex (VOR)**

3.2.1 **SCCs**

The VOR evolved to provide compensatory eye movements during movements of the head. It consists of inertial linear and rotational acceleration sensors, neural connections, and extra-ocular muscles as effectors. The SCCs are most sensitive to brief

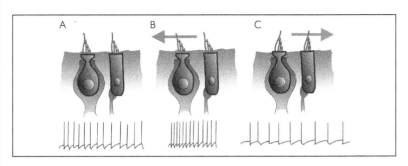

Figure 3.1 Stereocilia deflection modifies spontaneous activity. A. Spontaneous activity at rest (resting discharge); figures in the lower row symbolize the spikes of the action potentials. B. Deflection in the direction of the tallest stereocilia increases the spontaneous activity. C. Deflection in the opposite direction inhibits discharge.

angular accelerations (rotational VOR); otolithic organs measure linear accelerations (translational VOR during static tilts and translational head movements). The rotational VOR produces compensatory eye movements during head rotations, i.e. in order to retain the point of fixation, the eyes move relative to the head in the opposite direction. The effectiveness of the reflex is usually referred to as 'gain', which is defined as the ratio of eye velocity divided by head velocity. The horizontal rotational VOR has a velocity gain of close to one at medium and high head accelerations. The most dominant inputs for driving rotational VOR come from the SCCs, but the otolithic organs can also sense tangential and centrifugal forces during rotational head accelerations in all directions.

Compensatory eye movements have to be fast (Figure 3.2). During walking, every footfall causes sudden perturbations of the spine that are transmitted to the head. These movements have a frequency of 0.5 to 5 Hz, which means that up to five small amplitude, instantaneous head movements may occur during one second. During running, the frequency of skull vibrations may even reach 20 Hz. Retinal slip of images can also generate visually mediated eye movements by a cortical mechanism, with latencies longer than 70 milliseconds. This so-called smooth pursuit system is only effective during slow head movements or when gazing at a slowly moving object. In case of bilateral SCC dysfunction, unnoticed retinal slips drive eye movements. However during fast, unanticipated head perturbations, this system soon saturates, and visual acuity decreases. Patients note retinal slip as movements of the visual field (oscillopsia). This can be disturbing in everyday life. Patients with missing bilateral vestibular function, for instance, may find it difficult to recognize faces during normal walking on the street.

Compensatory eye movements must start almost simultaneously with head movements, i.e. with latencies shorter than 15 milliseconds, and they have to start in the correct direction: depending on the starting position of the eyeballs, different compensatory movements may be necessary. To be really fast and make lengthy three-dimensional calculations unnecessary, the breakdown of the three-dimensional space into individual planes occurs in the labyrinth. The canals, these toroidal angular accelerometers, are

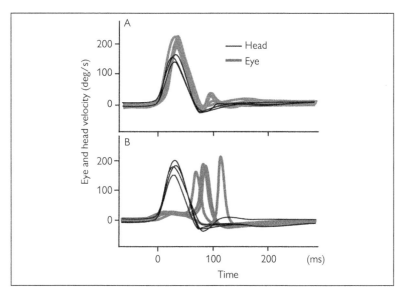

Figure 3.2 Compensatory eye movements during head rotations as measured with high-speed video-oculography. The head movements and the compensatory eye movements during fixation occur in the opposite direction (here superimposed upward in the same direction for better comparison). A. Normal. B. Decreased canal function (low gain); note the late compensatory saccades, with a latency of approx. 100 milliseconds. deg/s: degrees/second; ms: milliseconds.

positioned in the three perpendicular planes of the three dimensions, and each of them evokes compensatory eye movements in its own plane. During head rotations in the plane of the canal, the endolymph exerts pressure on the cupulae because of its inertia, and the resulting displacement of the cupulae is approximately proportional to head **velocity**. In this way, the SCCs supply the brain with head velocity signals.

The pulling directions of the muscles are arranged in a way that **the axis** of compensatory eye movements is aligned in the same direction in space as the axis of the SCC (Figure 3.3). Thus, the eye movements occur in the plane of the excited SCC, independently of eye position. This principle of 'SCC-fixed coordinate system' is important when discussing pathologies—dysfunction of one peripheral vestibular organ causes eye movements (nystagmus) with a fixed axis, and this axis is fixed to the SCCs, not to the eyeball. Gaze-dependent change of the axis orientation of the nystagmus is a central sign.

The 'anterior' canals are also called 'superior' in the literature; 'inferior' is also used for the 'posterior' canal. Concerning different disease entities, the nomenclature is not always consistent (such as 'superior' canal dehiscence but 'posterior' canal canalolithiasis instead of 'inferior'), so in this book we shall use the different names as synonyms.

The left anterior (LA) canal is approximately coplanar with the right posterior (RP) SCC (LARP plane), the right anterior (RA) SCC shares the plane with the left posterior (LP) canal (RALP plane) (Figure 3.4). The two horizontal SCCs are approximately

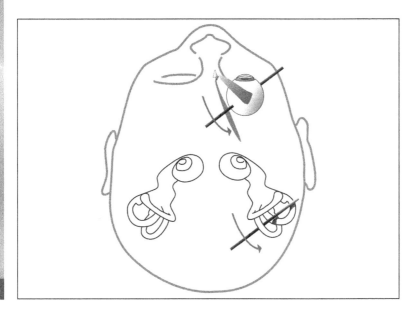

Figure 3.3 Sensitivity axis of the right posterior (RP) SCC. Explanation: see text.

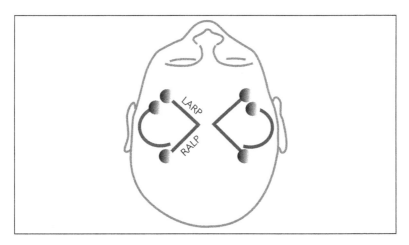

Figure 3.4 Diagonal vertical canal planes. LA: left anterior; RP: right posterior; RA: right anterior; LP: left posterior.

horizontal in upright position. The coplanar SCCs work as reciprocal pairs in a push-pull fashion. Whereas head rotation excites one SCC on one side, the same movement inhibits its coplanar counterpart on the other side.

3.2.2 Otolith organs

Otoconia, complex calcium carbonate biominerals, are embedded in a gelatinous layer over the utricular and saccular hair cells. The endolymphatic fluid has a very low calcium concentration, and the on-site otolith formation is a tightly regulated, active process. Due to a special fibrous structure, the otoconial membrane is compliant to shearing but not to compressional forces. During translational head movements, the otoconia help to stabilize the image on the retina via the translational VOR. Because of the equivalence of linear acceleration and the gravito-inertial force, otoliths are also sensitive to gravity. The otolith signals, converging with SCC signals, contribute to detect static head tilts relative to the gravity vector. During sustained lateral tilt of the head, this static otolith-ocular reflex produces ocular counter-rolling due to the head position change (compensating for approximately 10% of head roll).

The utricular and saccular maculae are curved structures; therefore, they sense linear accelerations in many different directions. The saccular macula is positioned in an almost vertical position; therefore, it is most sensitive to vertical up-and-down translations of the head. The utricular macula lies almost horizontally on the floor of the utricle; it is most sensitive to lateral or fore-aft tilts and side-to-side translations. Both otolith organs are curved and therefore overlapping in these functions. One-sided loss of utricular function causes a dominance of activity coming from the intact side. This is interpreted by the central nervous system (CNS) as a sideways tilt of the head to the intact side, probably because of the predominance of afferents arising from the medial aspect of the (intact) utriculus, which is sensitive to accelerations produced by ipsilateral tilts (see also ocular tilt reaction (OTR), Chapter 5). Modulation of saccular afferent activity causes change of tonus in muscles responsible for posture. According to theory, these saccular afferents may suddenly change their activity due to labyrinthine hydrops (Ménière's disease; MD) and then patients may fall without warning (Tumarkin's otolithic crisis). Both the utricular and the saccular macula can be simulated by loud sound and bone conducted vibrations; this is the basis of vestibular evoked potential testing (see Figure 3.5).

3.2.3 Vestibular nerve and nuclei

The vestibular nerve has two branches; the superior branch innervates the horizontal canal, the superior canal ampulla, the utricular macula, and the hook region of the saccular macula; the inferior branch innervates the inferior canal ampulla and the shank region of the saccular macula (Figure 3.6). Loss of function may occur with different patterns according to this anatomical division. In mammals, two classes of afferent neurons have been described. Regular afferents from the peripheral zones of the cupulae and maculae fire tonically with 50 to 100 spikes/second at rest, with very little variation of the resting rate. In contrast, irregular afferents from the central zones of the epithelium fire irregularly; they have a wider range of spontaneous rates

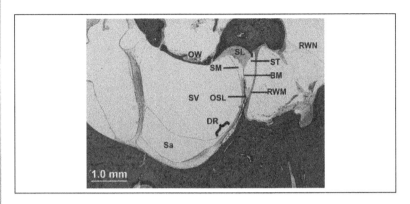

Figure 3.5 Histological section through the labyrinth showing the relation of stapes movements to the saccular macula. The close relationship between the stapes footplate (here seen in the oval window (OW)) makes the sacculus (Sa) and the utricular macula (running vertically, left from the sacculus) especially sensitive to sound. BM: Organ of Corti on the basilar membrane; RWM: round window membrane; OSL: osseous spiral lamina; SV: scala vestibuli; ST: scala tympani; RWN: round window niche; DR: ductus reuniens; SL: spiral ligament. Reprinted with permission from Li PM, Wang H, Northrop C, Merchant SN, Nadol JB Jr. (2007) Anatomy of the round window and hook region of the cochlea with implications for cochlear implantation and other endocochlear surgical procedures. *Otol Neurotol*. Aug;28(5):641–8. © Wolters Kluwer Health, 2007. See also colour plate section.

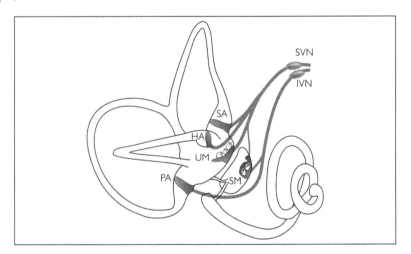

Figure 3.6 Superior and inferior vestibular nerve. SVN: superior vestibular nerve; IVN: inferior vestibular nerve; SA: superior ampulla; HA: horizontal ampulla; UM: utricular macula; PA: posterior ampulla; SM: saccular macula.

than do regular fibres. Their response to a given stimulus shows phasic behaviour; it is transient and follows the **rate of change** of the stimulus rather than the stimulus profile. These units may be very sensitive to vestibular stimuli. As we mentioned, hair cells are also of two types, I and II, but the two types do not correspond directly to the two afferent nerve cell populations. The relevance of the different hair cell and neuron groups is not fully understood. The clinical significance of the two classes is that irregular afferents are more sensitive to vibration, galvanic stimulation, and to the toxic effects of gentamicin.

In the resting state, vestibular hair cells constantly leak neurotransmitter, causing a spontaneous firing of the vestibular afferent fibres with a rate of approximately 90 spikes/second. When the head is upright and not moving, corresponding neurons in the vestibular ganglia on both sides and in both left and right vestibular nuclei have equal spontaneous firing rates. Up- and down-modulation of this spontaneous activity by excitation or inhibition of hair cells causes an asymmetry in the vestibular nuclei in the brainstem, which is interpreted as acceleration to one side. In the case of unilateral vestibular loss, the remaining other side may supply bidirectional information about acceleration, provided the acceleration into the inhibitory direction does not drive the afferent firing rate into inhibitory cut-off (in which case the spike frequency of 90 spikes/second decreases to zero).

3.2.4 Generation of eye movements

During rotations and translations of the head and also during movements of images on the retina, the eyes move to and fro repetitively. The slow phase is the primary component, initiated by the physiological or pathological inputs of the vestibular organs or retinal slippage; the compensatory quick phase resets the eyes into their working range. By convention, the nystagmus direction is named according to the direction of the quick phases. Sustained pathologic asymmetry of activity between canal pairs causes spontaneous nystagmus in the plane of these canals. If more canals are affected, the axis of the resulting nystagmus corresponds to the vectorial sum of the individual components.

During rotational head acceleration to the right in darkness while upright, the following events in the horizontal SCCs lead to the nystagmus (right panel, Figure 3.7):

- Because of inertia, endolymph moves to the left with respect to the head (on the right side in the direction of the cupula; on the left side away from it).
- The cupulae are deflected, and the hair cell depolarization causes transmitter release.
- Discharge of the primary afferents on the right increases and excites neurons in the right vestibular nucleus; on the left side, the discharge decreases, leading to inhibition of the ipsilateral vestibular nucleus neurons.
- Asymmetrical vestibular tone initiates the slow phase of the nystagmus towards the inhibited side (to the left side in this example).
- A quick resetting eye movement follows into the opposite (right) direction (not shown).

During head acceleration to the right, inhibitory neurons in the left vestibular nuclei decrease the activity they exert on the right side, thereby **disinhibiting** the neurons on the right side through commissural connections. This increases asymmetry and makes the system more sensitive. From a clinical point of view, the take home message is that, during head acceleration to the right, spontaneous activity on the

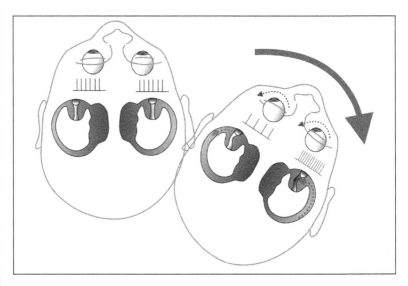

Figure 3.7 Vestibular asymmetry generates nystagmus slow phase. Left panel: spontaneous activity at rest; right panel: asymmetry due to acceleration to the right (arrow). The slow phase of the nystagmus is the primary, compensatory phase, directed to the left. Dotted arrows: endolymph movements and the slow phase of the nystagmus.

right side increases. This causes an eye movement with a slow phase to the left and a fast phase to the right. Therefore, in the case of a spontaneous nystagmus with a quick phase to the right, vestibular asymmetry with a higher activity on the right side may be assumed. This can be caused by either hypofunction on the left side (as in vestibular neuritis (VN)), or increased activity (excitation) on the right (as sometimes occurs in MD).

In the SCC, during a rotatory acceleration to the contralateral side, the spontaneous activity decays from 90 spikes/second to zero around velocities well below 200 degrees/second ('inhibitory cut-off'). However, in the excitatory direction, the activity increases linearly for rotational velocities up to 400 degrees/second. This means that, at high velocities, eye movements are driven by the SCCs on the side **ipsilateral** to the rotation. The head impulse test (HIT) is based on this principle.

Vestibular centres receive inputs from proprioceptive sensors in the limbs via gravity receptors in major blood vessels and abdominal viscera; also, visual cues help orientation in cases of bilateral vestibular loss. Secondary neurons in the vestibular nuclei send information about head movements to the ocular motor nuclei, to cervical spinal motor neurons, to lower spinal motor neurons, and to the cerebellum. Vestibular inputs are also transmitted to autonomic centres and to the cortex. Interruptions along the ascending or descending central vestibular pathways lead to impaired vestibulo-ocular and vestibulo-spinal functions.

3.3 Brainstem mechanisms assisting eye movements

3.3.1 Vestibular, optokinetic eye movements and velocity storage

The VOR has an optimal frequency range of function in response to brief accelerations and high frequency motion of the head. At sustained velocites, the cupula quickly returns to its neutral position; therefore, at lower frequencies of head movements, the measurement accuracy of the SCCs declines. The optokinetic system evolved as a synergistic system to improve gaze stabilization through retino-ocular reflexes with latencies of 100 milliseconds. It is optimized for gaze stabilization during head movements with low frequency, full-field visual stimuli and is closely related to the mechanisms generating smooth pursuit. Because of its polysynaptic character, it needs time to calculate the retinal slip and the required compensatory eye movements. With increasing frequencies (above 0.1-1 Hz), it saturates, retinal slip increases, and the system needs the input of the peripheral vestibular organs to generate compensatory eye movements with sufficiently short latency for visual stability. There is also a system of neural circuits in the brainstem that bridges the frequency spectrum between the two systems by extending the sensitivity of the VOR into the low frequency range. This so-called 'velocity storage mechanism' prolongs the effects of the canal signal, so the nystagmus lasts longer than the time required for the cupula to return to its neutral position. This storage mechanism can be loaded by increased afferent frequency due to acceleration in the ipsilateral direction. When the acceleration subsides, the system discharges, prolonging nystagmus and angular self-motion perception. The velocity storage mechanism also has an important clinical significance. In the case of unilateral vestibular loss, it is possible to asymmetrically load the mechanism by head shaking. In the case of a unilateral peripheral lesion, ipsilesional head turn does not load the integrator; this is achieved with every turn to the healthy side. In this direction, ipsilesional inhibitory signals are also missing. Therefore, after spontaneous nystagmus has subsided, it is possible to demonstrate one-sided peripheral vestibular loss by observing head-shaking nystagmus (more precisely: nystagmus after head shaking) under Frenzel's lenses after passively rotating the subject's head horizontally to and fro 20–25 times. Velocity storage is also responsible for the post-rotatory nystagmus after sustained constant acceleration.

3.3.2 Velocity-to-position integrator

Similar to velocity storage, there are other neuronal networks in the brainstem which modify commands generated by the vestibular centres. The velocity-to-position integrator estimates the eye position and counteracts the elastic properties of the eye muscles during gaze. By increasing the activity of the ocular muscles, which pull the eyes in the direction of the slow phase, it helps to diminish the sliding back of the eyeballs into primary gaze position. This circuit has clinical significance when spontaneous nystagmus is present. In the case of peripheral vestibular asymmetry, the brain tries to minimize the slow-phase drift of the eyes and the nystagmus by partially shutting down the velocity-to-position integrator, which ensures the eyes cannot be held in the direction of eccentric gaze and so drift back into the middle position. This is why the intensity of the spontaneous 'peripheral-type' nystagmus changes with gaze direction. When the eyes look in the direction of the slow phase, drifting back into the middle diminishes the velocity of the nystagmus; looking in the direction of the fast phase causes an addition of the drift and slow phase velocity, making the nystagmus faster and more frequent ('Alexander's law'). In cases of mild peripheral asymmetry, spontaneous nystagmus may manifest itself only during gaze in the direction of the fast phase (i.e. away from the lesioned side). This has to be differentiated from gaze-evoked nystagmus, which is a frequent central sign in cerebellar lesions and changes its direction depending on gaze. Since it is a function of the cerebellum to improve the performance of the integrator, cerebellar lesions may cause the integrator to be leaky. In these cases, the patient is not able to hold gaze in an eccentric position, leading to centripetal drift and centrifugal compensatory quick phases. Direction-changing nystagmus may be present unilaterally, that is, only during gaze in one direction (e.g. towards the side of lesion in cerebellar stroke). In these cases it is coarse and can be seen without Frenzel's goggles; the same cannot be said about peripheral spontaneous nystagmus, which is so weak as to be seen only during gaze towards the fast phase of the nystagmus.

3.4 **Blood supply**

From a clinical point of view, three arteries are the most important (Figure 3.8).

3.4.1 PICA

The PICAs originate usually from the vertebral arteries. The common trunk of the PICA gives rise to a medial branch and a lateral branch. The medial PICA supplies the inferior vermis of the cerebellum, including the nodulus and uvula, and the inferior

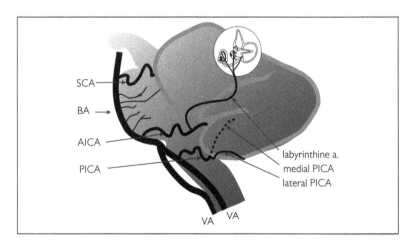

Figure 3.8 Posterior circulation. VA: vertebral arteries; PICA: posterior inferior cerebellar artery; AICA: anterior inferior cerebellar artery; BA: basilar artery; SCA: superior cerebellar artery; a: artery.

cerebellar hemisphere. The nodulus modulates the VOR and is closely connected to the vestibular nucleus and labyrinth. Because of all this, infarcts limited to the medial PICA may present as purely vestibular syndromes with severe vertigo, nausea, vomiting, and postural instability. The lateral PICA usually supplies the caudal portion of the lateral cerebellar hemisphere, which is involved in limb coordination.

3.4.2 AICA

The AICA originates in most cases from the lower half of the BA. The AICA is an important artery for vascular supply to the peripheral and central vestibular structures. The internal auditory artery is usually a branch of the AICA and supplies the VIII nerve, the cochlea, and the vestibular labyrinth. Since the AICA always supplies the lateral pontine tegmentum and the middle cerebellar peduncle, AICA territory infarcts usually involve the brainstem and are almost never limited to the cerebellum itself, whereas infarcts in the territory of the PICA or SCA usually involve only the cerebellum. The most common pattern of vestibular dysfunction in AICA territory infarction is a **combination** of peripheral (i.e. unilateral canal paresis leading to a pathological horizontal HIT (hHIT)), and central ocular motor or vestibular signs (i.e. asymmetrically impaired smooth pursuit, bidirectional gaze-evoked nystagmus or impaired modulation of the vestibular responses using visual input).

3.4.3 SCA

Since the superior cerebellum supplied by the SCA (branching from the upper part of the BA) does not have significant vestibular connections, cerebellar infarction in the SCA rarely causes rotating vertigo. Lateral SCA territory cerebellar infarction is characterized by dizziness, nausea, unsteadiness, mild truncal ataxia, and severe limb ataxia; medial SCA territory cerebellar infarction typically presents with severe gait ataxia with sudden falls or severe veering. Prominent body lateropulsion in isolated medial SCA territory cerebellar infarction may be explained by involvement of the rostral vermis, which is related predominantly to gait, muscle tone, and postural control.

3.5 **Unilateral vestibular loss**

Sudden unilateral loss of function causes static and dynamic disturbances. Static dysfunction occurs in the absence of head movements. Asymmetry of canal pairs causes nystagmus with the slow phase directed away from the intact ear. Asymmetry of the utricular nerve activity causes a complex pattern termed the OTR (see also Chapter 5). As mentioned, unilateral loss of utricular function is interpreted by the CNS as a sideways tilt of the head to the contralateral side (possibly because of the unopposed activity of the healthy utriculus). Since the patient has the feeling of head tilt towards the intact side, the reflexes try to compensate this, and the OTR occurs. It consists of a head tilt toward the side of the lesion, skew-deviation (disconjugate vertical deviation of the eyes, with the ipsilesional eye depressed and the other elevated), and ocular counter-rolling (with the upper poles of the eyes rotated toward the side of the lesion, i.e. the upper eye intorts and the lower eye extorts). This torsional ocular tonic deviation may also lead to nystagmus in the contra-torsional direction. A similar reaction may occur in lesions of the vestibular nuclei. Depending on the nuclei affected, cerebellar lesions may lead to contralesional or ipsilesional OTR. Since utricular projections cross the midline and ascend in the medial longitudinal fasciculus, partial or complete OTR caused by lesions of the ascending otolithic pathways rostral to the pontine level is contraversive, whereas lesions caudal to the pons (e.g. affecting the vestibular nuclei) lead to ipsiversive OTR.

3.5.1 Vestibular compensation

Neural recordings in animals recovering from unilateral vestibular loss show that central compensation depends on the restoration of normal spontaneous neural activity in the ipsilesional vestibular nucleus, thereby rebalancing activity of the left and right vestibular nuclei. After this rebalancing occurs, static symptoms disappear. However, dynamic disturbances, such as diminished excitability, can be demonstrated by bedside and auxiliary vestibular examination techniques if the peripheral end-organ does not recover.

References and Further Reading

Baloh R. W. and Halmágyi G. M. (eds). (1996) Disorders of the vestibular system. Oxford University Press, New York.

Carey J. P. and Della Santina C. (2005) Principles of applied vestibular physiology. In: Cummings C. W. (ed). Cummings Otolaryngology Head and Neck Surgery Vol IV, 4th edn Philadelphia, Elsevier Mosby. pp 3115–59.

Eatock R. A. and Songer J. E. (2011) Vestibular hair cells and afferents: two channels for head motion signals. *Annu Rev Neurosci.* **34**, 501–34.

Goldberg J. M., Wilson V. J., Cullen K. E. *et al.* (2012) The Vestibular System: A Sixth Sense. Oxford University Press.

Lee H. (2009) Neuro-otological aspects of cerebellar stroke syndrome. *J Clin Neurol.* **5**, 65–73.

Leigh R. J. and Zee D. S. (eds). (2006) The neurology of eye movements. Contemporary Neurology Series 4th edn Oxford University Press.

Li P.M., Wang H., Northrop C. *et al.* (2007) Anatomy of the round window and hook region of the cochlea with implications for cochlear implantation and other endocochlear surgical procedures. *Otol Neurotol.* **28**, 641–8.

Lundberg Y. W., Zhao X., Yamoah E. N. (2006) Assembly of the otoconia complex to the macular sensory epithelium of the vestibule. *Brain Res.* **1091**, 47–57.

Chapter 4

History of complaints as a diagnostic tool

Key points
• History taking in the dizzy patient should focus on the onset (abrupt vs gradually), duration (short vs long), and frequency of episodes (single vs recurrent), possible triggers, and accompanying symptoms (e.g. hearing loss).
• Identification of concomitant illnesses or drug intake may point to a non-vestibular disorder, whereas recurrent prodromal episodes and focal neurological symptoms make stroke more likely than vestibular neuritis (VN).
• In the presence of recent head/neck trauma and/or craniocervical pain, the examiner should aggressively search for vertebrobasilar dissection, although absence of pain or recent trauma does not exclude its presence.
• Vertebrobasilar stroke may present as isolated vertigo.
• The 'quality-of-symptom' approach is often non-diagnostic.
• Exacerbation of ongoing dizziness/vertigo with head movements does not allow a distinction between benign peripheral and dangerous central causes.
• Computed tomography (CT) scans of the posterior fossa detect stroke unreliably (with a sensitivity of < 40%) and should be replaced by magnetic resonance imaging (MRI).

4.1 Introduction

In the evaluation of the dizzy patient, detailed and structured history taking is essential, especially if intermittent episodes of dizziness or vertigo occur and the results of the clinical examination are unremarkable. Studies have suggested that, in up to 69–76% of dizzy patients, the diagnosis may be based on the history alone. Asking the 'right' questions is therefore crucial in making the correct diagnosis. History taking is often complicated by imprecise descriptions of complaints by the patients (was it spinning or sway, or did the patient instead experience imbalance?) and variable use of terms as vertigo or dizziness by patients, general practitioners, and even neurotologists. In this chapter we will discuss the most relevant aspects of history taking in the dizzy patient and the ways in which they help distinguishing different underlying pathologies.

4.2 **Frequency of spells**

Whereas many patients with a first episode of (prolonged) dizziness or vertigo will present to the emergency department (ED), general practitioners and outpatient centres will instead be confronted with patients reporting episodic dizziness or vertigo. Initially, it remains unclear whether the first dizzy spell will be followed by subsequent spells. Therefore during or shortly after an ongoing first dizzy spell, the differential diagnosis is broader than with recurrent symptoms. Some disorders may strongly vary in their presentation, ranging from brief to prolonged recurrent episodes of dizziness to permanent complaints. Vestibular migraine (VM) is such a candidate and therefore is a frequent differential diagnosis. VN occurs typically once (or perhaps twice) in a lifetime, benign paroxysmal positional vertigo (BPPV) may exacerbate perhaps once or twice annually, and attacks of Menière's disease (MD) may manifest weekly or even several times per week. Undoubtedly, benign entities are more frequent among recurrent symptoms. However, as we shall see, sometimes they signal more dangerous causes. Therefore, irrespective of whether these complaints are recurrent, dangerous and potentially life-threatening causes must be distinguished from more benign and self-limiting diseases.

4.2.1 **First episode of dizziness or vertigo**

When patients with a single episode of dizziness or vertigo present to the clinician, the dizzy spell may have already ceased or may still be ongoing. If the dizzy spell has already ended, or the patient has no complaints when completely motionless, provocatory tests may be applied to unmask BPPV. The differential diagnosis of a first dizzy spell is broad and strongly depends on symptom duration. It cuts across organ systems, including (transient) vestibular, cardiovascular, cerebrovascular, haematological, and metabolic disorders. Potentially dangerous first episodes of dizziness include transient ischaemic attack (TIA), vertebrobasilar stroke, drug intoxication, and cardiac arrhythmia. Exclusion of such possibly life-threatening causes is a priority.

4.2.2 **Recurrent dizziness/vertigo**

Episodic dizzy spells are encountered in a large range of disorders and may be mandatory to fulfil the diagnostic criteria, as for example in VM or MD. In other conditions, early treatment—e.g. for a first episode of BPPV—can prevent future spells. Patients with incomplete central compensation of a unilateral vestibular deficit tend to present with recurrent dizziness or vertigo in situations where the vestibular system is challenged, e.g. during rapid head movements. Recurrent dizzy spells may be related to both benign self-limited disorders such as BPPV, VM, or panic attacks, but dangerous, potentially life-threatening disorders, such as recurrent cardiac arrhythmia, hypoglycaemia, or vertebrobasilar TIA, may also be possible.

4.2.3 **Chronic dizziness/vertigo**

There is no consensus definition about the minimal duration of complaints to fulfil the criteria of **chronic** dizziness or vertigo. From a practical point of view, most patients with **chronic** dizziness/vertigo will report persistent symptoms over weeks to months. They often remain vague in their symptom description, and focused history taking for triggers and relieving factors is rarely helpful. Reported increase of complaints due to head motion is unspecific and does not distinguish peripheral from central causes. Potential diagnoses include VM, vestibular schwannoma (VS), bilateral vestibular deficits, severe polyneuropathy, and drug intoxication.

4.3 Episode duration—short vs long

Knowing the duration of a dizzy spell is very useful in the differential diagnosis, as most disorders present with a characteristic duration of single episodes. For example, vestibular paroxysmia lasts for only fractions of seconds. Provoked BPPV attacks last 15 to 30 seconds (after an acute phase of more intensive initial dizziness for hours or days), panic attacks subside after 10 to 20 minutes, attacks in MD typically last a maximum of two to three hours, and dizziness/vertigo due to VN or cerebellar stroke exceeds 24–48 hours. The range of duration typically encountered for the most frequent causes of dizziness/vertigo is illustrated in Figure 4.1. Whereas the majority of patients with VM have spells in the range of minutes to hours, 27% experience episodes lasting more than a day, which is relevant in the differential diagnosis of the acute vestibular syndrome (AVS; lasting >24 hours per definition). When asking about the duration of the dizzy spell, it is important to realize that, after cessation of intensive spinning or veering motion (e.g. as in BPPV), patients may still feel unsteady for hours to days before complaints stop completely. It is the duration of the intensive dizziness/vertigo that is considered here.

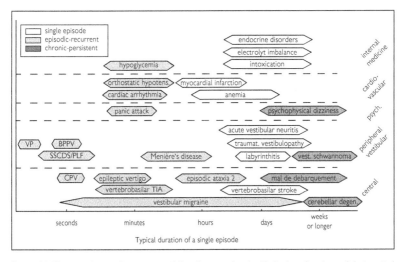

Figure 4.1 The most frequently encountered disorders associated with dizziness/vertigo and their typical range of symptom duration. The most frequently encountered disorders include vestibular, central, psychiatric, internal medicine, and cardiovascular diseases. Single or recurrent dizzy spells are distinguished from chronic dizziness/vertigo. CPV: central positional vertigo; PLF: perilymph fistula; SSCDS: superior semicircular canal dehiscence syndrome; VP: vestibular paroxysmia.

4.4 **Triggers**

Factors triggering recurrent attacks of dizziness or vertigo represent a key source of diagnostic information. Head movements up or down, lying down, or turning in bed are characteristic triggers for BPPV, as standing up is for orthostatic hypotension. Loud sounds or manipulation of upper airway pressure such as with the Valsalva manoeuvre may cause vertigo in cases of semicircular canal dehiscence (SCCD). Pressure increase in the outer ear canal sometimes elicits a short dizziness spell in MD (Hennebert's sign) or with erosion of the horizontal semicircular canal (SSC) in chronic otitis media. In case of persistent positional nystagmus, a central cause such as a posterior fossa tumour or Arnold-Chiari Type I malformation must be searched for. Following quickly moving objects with the eyes or suddenly losing the immediate reference system when entering wide, open spaces often may trigger dizziness (and panic) in patients with visual dominance of their sense of balance, whereas in patients with uni- or bilateral vestibular deficits, high-frequency head movements lead to blurring and dizziness. Triggers are typically absent in VM, MD, or cardiac arrhythmia and are scarce in dizziness preceding or accompanying an epileptic seizure. Overgeneralization of this rule to include AVS with persistent spontaneous nystagmus even when motionless, however, leads to the common misconception that exacerbation of symptoms with head movements (as with the Dix-Hallpike positional test for BPPV) predicts a peripheral cause. Specialists agree that AVS patients tend to be intolerant of head motion during the acute stage, regardless of the underlying localization as peripheral or central. Provocation testing is therefore not recommended in AVS due to its low diagnostic yield.

4.5 **Onset of symptoms**

For prolonged acute dizziness/vertigo as in AVS, an abrupt symptom onset favours a vascular cause, whereas more slowly evolving symptoms are encountered in VN or VM. In transient dizziness, however, abrupt symptom onset is frequently encountered (as in MD, BPPV, or vestibular paroxysmia (VP)) and is of little diagnostic help.

4.6 **Focal neurological symptoms, accompanying hearing loss or tinnitus**

Accompanying complaints as double vision, difficulty swallowing, slurred speech, limb weakness, or numbness strongly support a central cause of dizziness/vertigo—most likely stroke in the acute setting. However, their absence seems to be a relatively poor predictor of peripheral aetiology, as an isolated AVS is found in about 20–50% of cases. In chronic dizziness, the presence of afferent sensory impairments, e.g. due to severe polyneuropathy, spinal cord lesions, or vision loss, worsens complaints. Fluctuating hearing or frequently recurrent auditory symptoms with or without tinnitus point to a peripheral cause (i.e. MD) and sudden hearing loss to central localization in patients with dizziness/vertigo; auditory symptoms in AVS patients can and do result from inner ear ischaemia, often in association with frank posterior circulation infarction in the anterior inferior cerebellar artery (AICA) territory. Blurred vision, as it is related to retinal slip, may be noticed in patients with various kinds of nystagmus, but does not support a specific diagnosis. A short-lasting spinning or floating sensation may precede transient loss of consciousness (TLOC), as for example in the case of vasovagal syncope, seizures, or vertebrobasilar TIA, whereas other conditions with brief dizzy spells, such as BPPV, VP, MD, or VM, do not. The presence/absence of TLOC may therefore be useful in the differential diagnosis of short-lasting dizziness.

For patients with chronic or episodic dizziness, searching for signs of depression, anxiety disorders, or panic attacks is important, as psychiatric diagnoses and dizziness have been shown to be linked, resulting in an increased likelihood of dizziness in patients with depression, and vice versa. Presence of depression or anxiety disorders may suggest the use of behavioural therapy.

4.7 **Prodromal or accompanying symptoms**

Hearing loss worsening over days or weeks and pressure in the involved ear are typical prodromal symptoms in the Lermoyez variant of MD; hearing then improves during a vertigo attack. Otherwise, pressure in the ear, hearing loss, and tinnitus are typical accompanying symptoms in classical MD but with worsening hearing during the course of the disease; fluctuating hearing disappears, and permanent hearing loss develops. In other peripheral entities, the absence of accompanying symptoms is characteristic, such as in VN or BPPV, although, interestingly, with BPPV, patients sometimes feel pressure or 'movements' in the involved ear. Unilateral sensorineural hearing loss with permanent slight dizziness over months may indicate VS. Middle ear hearing loss with episodic vertigo occurs in the syndrome of 'a pathological third window of the labyrinth' (see Chapter 8).

Headache as an accompanying symptom may signify dangerous central pathologies but is more frequent in VM. **Craniocervical pain** may accompany dizziness/vertigo in posterior fossa strokes as a result of the stroke itself (mass effect or direct involvement of pain-sensitive structures) or of its underlying cause (e.g. vertebral artery dissection (VAD) or aneurysm). Occipital pain may be a red flag in meningitis. Note that occipital and cervical pain which is worse during the night and may even wake the patient from sleep should raise the possibility of aseptic meningitis in Lyme disease, which sometimes may be associated with dizziness.

Because migraine is a diagnostic consideration in almost any patient with dizziness/vertigo and headache, there is evidence that young patients with VAD and posterior fossa stroke may be at particularly high risk of being misdiagnosed with migraine. Unlike the gradually increasing headache that disappears within 24–48 hours typically encountered in migraine, craniocervical pain is of sudden onset, prolonged (i.e. lasting more than 72 hours) and severe in a majority of patients diagnosed with VAD. The absence of pain appears to be diagnostically inconclusive with regard to ruling out VAD; roughly one in four dissection patients presents without head or neck pain.

Transient dizziness, hearing loss, and/or tinnitus as a premonitory TIA can precede audio-vestibular loss due to AICA infarction in up to 42% of cases. Patients with sudden hearing loss were found to be at increased stroke risk. While a **single** episode of transient dizziness/vertigo within a few days prior to AVS presentation is probably non-specific (reported with high frequency in both VN and stroke), recurrent episodes lasting seconds to minutes over the preceding weeks or months may favour a cerebrovascular cause and have been reported in up to 29% of vertebrobasilar stroke patients.

4.8 **Type or quality of dizziness/vertigo**

Traditionally it has been taught that the **type** or **quality** of symptoms directs the subsequent diagnostic inquiry. In brief, the 'quality of symptoms approach' states that vertigo indicates a vestibular cause, presyncope a cardiovascular cause, disequilibrium a neurologic cause, and unspecific dizziness a psychiatric or metabolic cause. This approach, however, seems not to be evidence-based practice. A study carried out in the emergency medicine setting on over 300 consecutive patients with acute dizziness has shown the type of symptoms (dizziness vs vertigo vs disequilibrium vs presyncope) to be an imprecise metric—more than half of the patients were unable to reliably report which symptom type most accurately reflected their complaints (Newman-Toker et al 2007). More importantly, symptom quality does not appear to be a trustworthy predictor of underlying aetiology. It was shown that patients with unsteadiness as part of their symptom complex were at slightly higher risk of stroke, but vertigo vs other dizziness predicted stroke with equal likelihood. These shortcomings in describing the feeling of motion/unsteadiness may be associated with the patient's unfamiliarity with dizziness, the shortness of the spells (not giving the subject enough time to focus on symptom details), and distraction by associated symptoms, such as intensive nausea and vomiting. The clinician, therefore, should put more emphasis on the timing, triggers, and prodromal symptoms of the current episode, as discussed.

4.9 **Concurrent illnesses and medication use**

Whereas about 30% of patients with dizziness presenting to the ED have underlying neurotological disorders, dizziness/vertigo is related to non-vestibular problems in the majority of patients. When obtaining the medical history from the dizzy patient, one should therefore identify any major known, **concurrent illnesses** (e.g. multiple sclerosis (MS), HIV-AIDS, metastatic malignancy, severe malnutrition, major depression, diabetes) or **potentially-relevant exposures** (e.g. viral syndrome, ear surgery, bacterial otitis media, or ototoxic medications (especially aminoglycoside antibiotics)) in addition to assessing vascular risk factors. Persistent dizziness is a frequent side effect of many drugs, including neuro-modulatory substances (e.g. anti-depressants, anti-epileptics, and sedatives), diuretics, and antihypertensive drugs. While being most prominent in case of intoxication (e.g. with phenytoin, lithium, or carbamazepine), intake of a new drug or increasing the dosage of an established substance may lead as well to drug-related dizziness or vertigo (e.g. with gabapentin).

4.10 **Proportionality of complaints**

Proportionality of dizziness, neurovegetative, and gait/postural symptoms has sometimes been cited by experts as typical of peripheral vestibular disorders, whereas central syndromes are said to occasionally be associated with disproportionate symptoms (e.g. severe gait impairment with a mild subjective sense of dizziness or vertigo).

Authors of uncontrolled case reports and small case series hypothesized that the presence of vomiting or imbalance/gait unsteadiness out of proportion to the degree of dizziness or nystagmus may be a marker for brainstem or cerebellar pathology, including stroke.

4.11 Age

With advancing age, BPPV, stroke, cardiac arrhythmia, or drug intoxication are more frequently encountered. Though age is a known risk factor for stroke, it should still be considered in younger patients. In the largest prospective study of AVS patients, 25% with ischaemic stroke (mostly due to VAD or occlusion) were under 50 years of age. VM may start in the second or third decade of life and vasovagal (pre)syncope with prodromal dizziness is frequently observed in the young.

4.12 Recent trauma

BPPV has been associated with preceding head trauma. Trauma or sudden pressure increase may open a third window on the labyrinth (causing fluctuating vertigo) or involve the otic capsule in temporal bone fractures (bringing about a permanent vestibular deafferentation).

Recent head or neck **trauma** is a known risk factor for VAD, making its occurrence about four times more likely in case of minor trauma. Since VAD is a known cause of central AVS, a history of trauma should spark concern for underlying dissection. However, roughly half of symptomatic VADs occur **without** an identifiable history of trauma, so the absence of trauma is insufficient to exclude the diagnostic possibility of VAD. Traumatic epidural or subdural hematoma is also a diagnostic consideration in case of posttraumatic dizziness and can be readily identified by head CT.

4.13 Quality of life assessment

Recurrent episodic or chronic dizziness/vertigo may severely impact the patient's quality of life and daily activities and may result in isolation, dependence on others, and depression. Depending on the degree of central compensation and on the awareness of the patient, impairments due to residual vestibular hypofunction after VN may be perceived differently among affected individuals. When taking the history in such patients, impairments in the quality of life should be searched for, as their presence may underline the need for appropriate treatment, possibly including physical therapy, psychological counselling (with a focus on coping strategies), and medication (e.g. anti-depressants).

4.14 Common misconceptions in the assessment of the dizzy patient

In the evaluation of the dizzy patient, the clinician is faced with several misconceptions about the interpretation of findings. As a result, the examiner might associate certain findings falsely with more benign disorders, delaying or even preventing the initiation of more aggressive diagnostics and appropriate treatment (Stanton *et al* 2007). The most frequently encountered misconceptions are:

1) 'Isolated dizziness makes the diagnosis of stroke unlikely and favours a benign peripheral cause.' This assumption is not justified, as up to 50% of patients with central AVS may present with isolated dizziness/vertigo ('pseudoneuritis'), closely mimicking acute peripheral vestibulopathy.

2) 'Defining the type of symptoms ("quality-of-symptom" approach) can be used to distinguish dangerous central from more benign, self-limited peripheral aetiologies.' This approach, although it is classical teaching and common practice, has been shown to be of little value in differential diagnosis, as patients are imprecise and inconsistent in reporting the quality of their complaints, and either dizziness or vertigo may be the presenting feature in many underlying diagnoses as cardiac arrhythmia, BPPV, or cerebellar stroke.

3) 'Ongoing prolonged dizziness/vertigo that exacerbates with head movements points towards a benign peripheral cause.' Whereas in BPPV symptoms are triggered (and not exacerbated), patients with prolonged dizziness/vertigo will experience an increase in complaints when applying head movements independently from the underlying cause.

4) 'Negative CT scan of the brain rules out ischaemic stroke.' Sensitivity of CT for detecting ischaemic stroke in the posterior fossa is below 40%, and even early diffusion-weighted MRI can be negative within the first 24–48 hours in up to 20% of cases.

References and Further Reading

Kerber K. A. (2009) Vertigo and dizziness in the emergency department. *Emerg Med Clin North Am.* **27**, 39–50.

Newman-Toker D. E., Cannon L. M., Stofferahn M. E. *et al.* (2007) Imprecision in patient reports of dizziness symptom quality: a cross-sectional study conducted in an acute care setting. *Mayo Clin Proc.* **82**, 1329–40.

Stanton V. A., Hsieh Y. H., Camargo C.A. Jr *et al.* (2007) Overreliance on symptom quality in diagnosing dizziness: results of a multicenter survey of emergency physicians. *Mayo Clin Proc.* **82**, 1319–28.

Tusa R. J. (2010) Bedside assessment of the dizzy patient. In: Eggers S. D Z., Zee D. S. (eds). Vertigo and Imbalance: Clinical Neurophysiology of the Vestibular System. Handbook of Clinical Neurophysiology, Vol. 9. Elsevier B.V. pp. 43–58.

Chapter 5

Examination methods

Key points

- The aim of the vestibular examination is to search for static and dynamic vestibular dysfunctions and to assign these to central or peripheral pathologies.
- Bedside testing (ocular motor and other neurological signs) during an acute attack of vertigo may yield invaluable information.
- The head impulse test (HIT) assesses the vestibulo-ocular reflex (VOR) in its physiological working range.
- The utricle and saccule may be stimulated by air-conducted and bone-conducted vibrations.
- The saccule has neural connections to the ipsilateral sternocleidomastoid muscle, and the utricle projects strongly to contralateral ocular muscles. By choosing the corresponding electrode montage to record myogenic electrical activity elicited by short vibrations, it is possible to test the saccular (vestibulo-collic) and the utricular (vestibulo-ocular) reflex separately.
- Endolymphatic hydrops can be detected by non-invasive electrocochleography (Ecochg), thereby aiding the differential diagnosis of Menière's disease (MD), especially before considering ablating procedures such as intratympanic gentamicin instillation.

5.1 Introduction

Vestibular dysfunction may cause static and/or dynamic disturbances. Static dysfunction occurs upon sudden collapse of unilateral spontaneous activity leading to vestibular tone asymmetry in the brainstem vestibular nuclei. This asymmetry expresses itself by signs such as spontaneous nystagmus, which, although transient, may supply invaluable information if carefully documented. With time, even if peripheral vestibular activity does not recover on the lesioned side, central compensatory mechanisms reinstate symmetry. In this phase, the examination consists of an assessment of the dynamic performance of the system using physiological stimuli.

In this chapter we describe the components of bedside testing and several recently developed instrumental examinations. We do not discuss already established, sophisticated laboratory methods, such as electronystagmography combined with caloric testing or rotational testing, as these methods are well known and only available in specialized diagnostic units. However, we describe some new instrumental methods in order to help referrals and interpretation of test results.

5.2 **Bedside testing**

Bedside testing is most important in acute dizziness and vertigo. Its main goal is to search for vestibular asymmetry and to decide if this asymmetry is of peripheral or central origin. If there are signs of central vestibular dysfunction, this may raise the possibility of a more serious disorder. In Table 5.1, we list important bedside tests. The list is somewhat arbitrary; every examiner has to build his or her protocol, based on practice and personal experience. For instance, examination of smooth pursuit eye movements and optokinetic nystagmus are not included, because there is only insufficient evidence concerning their usefulness in the assessment of the acute vestibular syndrome (AVS; Tarnutzer *et al* 2011). Although it is well known that deficient smooth pursuit compensated by catch-up saccades is indicative of central oculomotor pathology, smaller cerebellar infarctions (extensive enough to elicit gaze-evoked nystagmus) rarely cause asymmetric smooth pursuit and optokinetic nystagmus (Lee *et al* 2006). Also, smooth pursuit loses its smoothness and becomes saccadic with age, which makes its evaluation difficult in the elderly. In particular, slightly saccadic **downward** pursuit may in fact be normal in this population.

5.2.1 **Vestibular-oculomotor examination**

Vestibular asymmetry elicited by activity difference of primary nerve fibres originating in the semicircular canals (SCCs) causes nystagmus in the plane of the affected canals; asymmetry of otolithic nerve fibres or their central vestibular pathways may cause an ocular tilt reaction (OTR), which consists of skew deviation (vertical misalignment of the eyes), ocular counter-rolling, and head tilt. The most important components of the

---

Table 5.1 Bedside tests

- Vestibular-oculomotor examination (search for vestibular asymmetry or central oculomotor disturbances)
  - Search for nystagmus
    - Search for spontaneous nystagmus
    - with fixation
    - without fixation
    - Search for gaze-evoked (direction-changing) nystagmus
  - Search for vertical misalignment of the eyes (cover test)
  - Provocation testing
    - Head shaking (if no spontaneous nystagmus)
    - Search for positional nystagmus (positional testing)
- Testing of the VOR (search for dynamic disturbances)
- Search for neurologic signs
- Otological examination
  - Otoscopy
  - Whisper test of hearing

vestibular-oculomotor evaluation in acutely dizzy patients are examination of spontaneous signs in gaze straight ahead (ocular misalignment and/or spontaneous nystagmus), searching for direction-changing nystagmus, and tests of provocation (head shaking, positional provocation).

5.2.1.1 Nystagmus

Vestibular nystagmus is a jerk nystagmus; it consists of repetitive, to and fro movements of the eyes initiated by a slow drift (slow phase) followed by a fast, compensatory phase. In clinical terms, nystagmus is described by the direction of the quick, corrective phase; however, it is the slow phase that is generated by the asymmetry in the primary vestibular afferents, which is in turn caused by the underlying disorder. Pendular nystagmus does not show this distinct two-phase pattern.

Nystagmus may be caused by disorders of the peripheral vestibular system, or by central disturbances of gaze-holding mechanisms and visual stabilization systems.

Search for spontaneous nystagmus is first carried out during fixation in the central position, then in 30-degree eccentric gaze angles. Next, this examination should be repeated, the eyes being observed under Frenzel's goggles to exclude the suppressive effect of visual fixation. Fixation may be prevented by other means as well, such as placing a white sheet close before the eyes and observing the unfixing gaze from above; or by a penlight shone in the eye, intermittently covering the other eye (the penlight test, Newman-Toker et al 2009). Expert opinion suggests that peripheral nystagmus increases when removing fixation. If the intensity of the nystagmus is similar both with and without fixation or even increases with fixation, this suggests dysfunction of the central fixation neural network.

Spontaneous peripheral vestibular nystagmus signalizes acute tonic asymmetry between the brainstem vestibular nuclei. It changes its intensity but not its direction as a function of gaze-direction (it is more intensive during gaze into the direction of the fast phase (see Chapter 3)). The plane of peripheral spontaneous nystagmus is a result of the vector summation of the activity difference between individual canal planes.

Central spontaneous nystagmus. Pure vertical (upbeat or downbeat) or torsional nystagmus is typically central. Downbeat nystagmus may be idiopathic or caused by cerebellar flocculus degeneration and lesions around the craniocervical junction, such as the Arnold-Chiari malformation. Less frequent causes are encephalitis, hydrocephalus, B_{12} deficiency, and lithium intoxication. Downbeat nystagmus is usually stronger on lateral gaze and downgaze. Upbeat nystagmus may occur with lesions of the dorsal upper medulla or of the midbrain (infarction, tumour, or multiple sclerosis) and is typically transient.

Gaze-evoked (direction-changing) nystagmus. Cerebellar or brainstem lesions cause a dysfunction of the velocity-to-position integrator, which helps to hold gaze in eccentric positions. When the integrator is leaky, the eyes drift back in the central position. Gaze-evoked nystagmus should be differentiated from physiological end-point nystagmus, which arises beyond lateral gaze angles of 30–40 degrees. Cerebellar infarction, for instance, causes direction-changing bidirectional gaze-evoked nystagmus with maximal intensity during gaze to the lesion side or direction-fixed unidirectional gaze-evoked nystagmus beating toward the side of the lesion (Lee et al 2006).

Periodic alternating nystagmus (PAN). PAN refers to a congenital or acquired spontaneous horizontal jerk nystagmus that reverses direction periodically. Lesions in the craniocervical junction, isolated infarction of the cerebellar nodulus, and cerebellar atrophy may lead to PAN.

Pendular nystagmus. Pendular nystagmus corresponds to back and forth eye oscillations without resetting quick phases. Acquired pendular nystagmus mainly occurs in multiple sclerosis (MS) and focal brainstem lesions and can be accompanied by palatal tremor in the latter case. Clinically, it leads to impaired visual fixation and oscillopsia.

Seesaw nystagmus. Elevation and intorsion of one eye and synchronous depression and extorsion of the other eye followed by reversal of these pendular or jerk movements result in 'seesaw'-like movements. This rare nystagmus typically occurs with lesions in the meso-diencephalic junction, as unilateral lesions of the interstitial nucleus of Cajal.

5.2.1.2 Misalignment of the eyes

Unilateral lesions of the otolith organs or their central vestibular pathways cause an OTR. The complete OTR consists of head tilt, conjugate binocular eye torsion, and skew deviation (vertical misalignment of the eyes). The basis of OTR is a vestigial labyrinthine righting reflex. In the case of a unilateral peripheral otolithic lesion, the unopposed activity of the intact contralateral side dominates. Therefore, unilateral peripheral vestibular dysfunction (otolithic deafferentation) causes a complete or, more often, partial OTR towards the side of the lesion (ipsilesional head tilt; a disconjugate deviation (skew deviation) of the eyes with an elevated pupil on the intact side and hypotropia (downward deviation) on the side of the lesion; and a static conjugate counter roll of the eyes, rolling the superior pole of each eye toward the side of the lesion). The head tilt and skew deviation are often absent, whereas static ocular torsion may be present for a longer time, even if with declining intensity. This conjugate ocular torsion towards the affected side may be measured with indirect ophthalmoscopy or fundus photography. Since the patients have the feeling that their head position is vertical in spite of the OTR, they offset a luminous line in an angle from the horizontal or vertical position if they are deprived of clues helping orientation (examination of subjective visual vertical or horizontal; see Section 5.3.4). Dysfunction of the central otolithic connections also causes skew deviation and OTR. Because of the crossing of the pathways approximately at the level of the vestibular nuclei, the OTR is ipsiversive with pontomedullary lesions (as with peripheral lesions), and contraversive with pontomesencephalic or more rostral lesions.

5.2.1.3 Provocation testing of the VOR

During provocation testing of the SCCs and the rotational VOR, the examiner elicits endolymph movements in the canals and interprets the resulting eye movements. This can be done by altering head position (if otolithic debris floats freely in the SCC as in benign paroxysmal positional vertigo (BPPV)), by fast, passive head movements (head shaking and impulsive testing), and by altering the density of the endolymph by thermal stimulations (caloric reaction). The endolymph may be moved by applying loud sounds, vibrations, or pressure to the ear canal if there is a dehiscence on one of the SCCs. It is also possible to provoke the vestibular system without eliciting endolymph movements: hyperventilation (possibly by the respiratory alkalosis and reduction of plasma pCO_2 and free Ca^{2+} concentration) sometimes induces nystagmus in cases of vestibular nerve compression (schwannoma), demyelination of its root entry zone, or with cerebellar pathologies.

Head shaking. If the vestibular asymmetry subsided and the spontaneous nystagmus disappeared, for some time it is possible to 'go back in time' and recall the short term, past history of vestibular asymmetry by head shaking. Passively rotating the subject's head horizontally to and fro 20–25 times loads the brainstem velocity storage circuits asymmetrically in the case of asymmetric peripheral vestibular excitability. Nystagmus should be observed under Frenzel's lenses after the vigorous head shaking, beating away from the affected side. This simple test is very useful when the patient visits the outpatient centre after his or her most serious symptoms have abated.

Positional testing. Normally, SCCs should only be excited by angular accelerations, but if otolithic debris enters them (canalolithiasis) or adheres to the cupulae (cupulolithiasis), this may sensitize them to gravity. The most important role of the positional testing is to demonstrate if that is indeed the case. The principle of examination is the following: in sitting (or supine) position, the debris gathers at the most inferior point of the SCCs. Then the head should be moved in a new position. If this occurs in the plane of the canal, the way before the debris will become free and the dislodged otoconia will move into the lowermost part of the SCC. The movements of the debris elicit nystagmus in the plane of the affected canal. Since the vertical canals are positioned in diagonal planes, the left posterior (LP) and right anterior (RA) canals (and the right posterior (RP) and left anterior (LA) ones) can be tested by the same diagonal head-hanging position (the so-called Dix-Hallpike position). In order to test the horizontal canals, the head should be positioned sideways, into the lateral positions, preferable from the face-up supine position. Positioning the patient from sitting in the supine position may elicit the so-called 'lying-down' nystagmus in horizontal canalolithiasis. The examiner should be aware that a slight peripheral horizontal-rotatory spontaneous nystagmus may be enhanced in lateral supine or in Dix-Hallpike positions and may thus be mistaken for a positional nystagmus.

Canalolithiasis produces transient nystagmus after a few seconds of latency, typically lasting less than 15 to 30 seconds; cupulolithiasis causes a more persistent, less intensive nystagmus reaction. With larger masses of debris and repeated manoeuvres, the accompanying motion sickness may exhaust the patient and even elicit vomiting, especially in cases of horizontal canalolithiasis. Relatively recently, the theory of short arm canalolithiasis has been suggested (see Chapter 12), when the Dix-Hallpike and lateral provoking positions do not elicit nystagmus but there is a strong trunk sway and even retropulsion when sitting up from the Dix-Hallpike position. The examiner should note these signs too, as well as the direction, intensity, and duration of nystagmus.

Positional nystagmus: central or peripheral? Positional nystagmus may also be caused by central pathologies. Cerebellar tumours and Arnold-Chiari syndrome may cause positional downbeat nystagmus; cerebellar infarction sometimes causes direction-changing laterally beating horizontal positional nystagmus, which may be seen in the lateral supine position. Tumours or haemorrhages in the dorsal vermis or in the cerebellum around the fourth ventricle may cause positional nystagmus and vertigo, which may be impossible to differentiate clinically from a peripheral positional nystagmus. Nystagmus lasting as long as the positional provocation, positional nystagmus without vertigo, and positional vomiting without nystagmus are presumably central signs (Büttner *et al* 1999).

Nystagmus induced by pressure, sound, or vibration. With SCC dehiscence, loud sounds, tragal pressure or the Valsalva manoeuvre may induce nystagmus in the plane of the affected canal, possibly because the pathological third window allows increased endolymph movements. Vibration applied on the mastoid may—similarly to the head-shaking nystagmus—unmask the central compensation of a past peripheral vestibular deficit by eliciting a vibration-induced nystagmus with the fast phase beating away from the affected side. Presumably, unilateral mastoid vibration stimulates the vestibular organs on both sides. This nystagmus should be observed under Frenzel's goggles.

Caloric testing. By eliciting thermal gradients and endolymph density changes, it is possible to stimulate the SCC in the low frequency range. Apparently, velocity and direction of caloric nystagmus depend not only on the absolute magnitude of vestibular activity on the stimulated side but also on asymmetry of activity (firing rate) between the left and right vestibular nuclei, most probably mediated centrally via brainstem commissural pathways (Aw *et al* 2000). If the slow phase velocity of the nystagmus evoked by warm and cold water or air irrigation is decreased on one side (canal paresis), this has localizing significance. If the slow phases to one side dominate on both sides during cold and warm irrigations (isolated directional preponderance), this is usually a transient, benign disorder. In a study by Halmagyi *et al* (2000), about half the patients with an isolated directional preponderance had peripheral vestibular dysfunction (MD or BPPV) and only approximately 5% had a central nervous system (CNS) lesion (apparent at the time the caloric test was done). The authors postulated that an isolated directional preponderance reflected a gain asymmetry between neurons in the medial vestibular nucleus on either side, caused by increased sensitivity on one side or by reduced sensitivity on the other, perhaps as an adaptive change in response to abnormal input.

HIT. (see Figure 5.1) The HIT assesses the VOR by its physiological output: the ability of the eyes to fixate a stationary target during brief, unexpected, high velocity, passive head rotations or translations. In the clinical routine, the HIT is carried out in the horizontal direction (horizontal HIT (hHIT)), to assess the horizontal canals. It is also possible to carry out a diagonal HIT to test the vertical canals in the left anterior right posterior (LARP) or (right anterior left posterior) RALP planes and head heaves to test the translational VOR. During these tests, compensatory eye movements with short latency or small amplitude may be difficult for the examiner to assess visually; however, there are commercially available systems consisting of fast infrared video goggles and acceleration sensors, which can be used to examine and document even separate vertical canal excitability.

The clinician carries out the head turns by hand; the subject is instructed to fixate a stationary target and to relax the neck muscles. However, the HIT should not be applied in patients with recent neck injury or chronic neck pain. To be applied correctly, the HIT has to fulfil several criteria, such as small amplitude (between 10–20 degrees to each side to prevent iatrogenic neck injury and allow for high accelerations) and high velocity. The latter is important to challenge the VOR faster than the range of the smooth pursuit and also to drive the afferents of the contralateral side into inhibitory

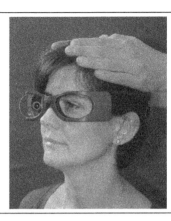

Figure 5.1 High-speed infrared video HIT (vHIT). The patient is instructed to fixate on a dot at a reference position straight ahead on a screen at a distance of approx. one metre. Head impulses are manually delivered by the examiner standing behind the subject.

cut-off (see Chapter 3), thereby making it possible to test the SCC almost exclusively unilaterally on the side to which the head is turning. In cases with unilateral dysfunction, velocities over 100–150 degrees/second are sufficient to demonstrate gain asymmetry. By carrying out the HIT in both the horizontal and vertical planes, separate canal pairs can be tested. Pathologically reduced SCC function is compensated by corrective saccades, which appear after the head turn ('overt' saccades) or during the head turn (hidden or 'covert' saccades) (Weber *et al* 2008). Overt saccades can easily be seen during bedside testing, even in spite of spontaneous nystagmus. For the analysis of covert saccades, high-speed infrared video goggles may be necessary.

These lightweight goggles, containing a high-speed infrared camera and acceleration sensors, make it possible to quantify the performance of each individual SCC to monitor changes of excitability in clinical settings. The excitability of the canals when measured by high-speed video goggles is expressed as reflex 'gain', the ratio of output to stimulus; that is, the ratio of eye velocity (or acceleration) divided by head velocity (or acceleration).

In normal individuals the gain of the horizontal VOR is close to unity over a broad range, up to velocities of 400 degrees/second. In cases of unilateral vestibular hypofunction, ipsilesional VOR gains decrease steeply with increasing head acceleration as the healthy contralateral side reaches its inhibitory cut-off. In case of unilateral hypofunction, the physiological disinhibition arriving from the side of the lesion is missing. Therefore, with unilateral vestibular loss, contralesional gains (during head accelerations to the healthy side) are also somewhat reduced. If the vestibular nerve has not been totally cut but just rendered partly dysfunctional amidst symptoms of sudden vestibular neuritis (VN; probably because of viral infection), ipsilesional gains are lower than those of normal values (but not as low as after complete deafferentation), and contralesional gains will be significantly reduced only above a certain head velocity (Figure 5.2).

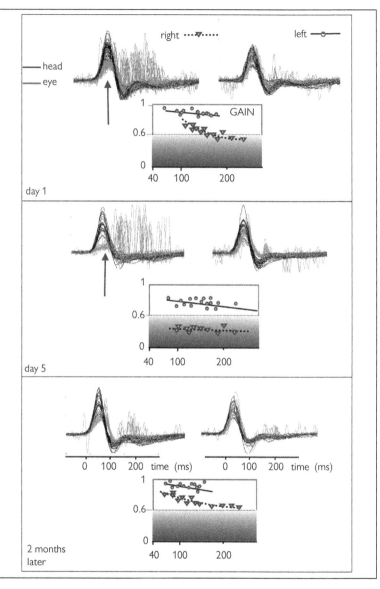

Figure 5.2 Clinical course of VN as monitored by horizontal vHIT. During the first week (day 1 and day 5), the hHIT showed a diminishing excitability of the right horizontal canal (upward vertical arrows). Two months later, the patient had no complaints, and the gain almost normalized.

Clinical significance. The HIT is important for examination of the AVS. Together with the search for gaze-evoked nystagmus and skew deviation, it is part of the HINTS (**H**ead **I**mpulse test, searching for direction-changing **N**ystagmus, and **T**est of **S**kew deviation) bedside test battery to differentiate dangerous central causes (mostly stroke) from benign peripheral causes (mostly VN). Since the quantitative HIT-measurement is fast and non-invasive, clinical progression, recovery, or effect of therapy (such as intratympanal gentamicin) can be monitored. After VN, if peripheral function does not recover, gain of VOR measured by vHIT remains decreased for a long time. HIT may be useful in diagnosing bilateral chronic vestibular insufficiency. Unlike caloric reaction, which is a very low frequency stimulus, this test assesses vestibular function in the physiological working range of the VOR.

5.2.2 Search for additional neurologic signs

The bedside examination of dizzy patients includes an orienting neurologic examination. Especially in acute dizziness, when collaboration of the patient is limited, it is important to search for subtle central neurologic signs beyond the oculomotor examination. Is facial nerve function normal? Is there hoarseness? If yes, vocal cord mobility (vagal nerve function) has to be assessed. Is there blurring of speech? Results of sensory testing for slight touch, pain, temperature, position sense, and vibration (face, arms, trunk and legs) may be informative. Hearing may be tested by the whisper test (whispered voice with the other ear finger-masked). Even during a vertigo attack, it is important to document the side and progression of fluctuating partial hearing loss (MD) or acute deafness (possible anterior inferior cerebellar artery (AICA)-infarction). Chronic partial symmetrical hearing loss is rarely relevant to vestibular diagnosis. Coordination should be tested in the sitting position (although it is also possible in the supine position if the patient cannot be moved, e.g. because of vomiting) by performing simple tasks, such as asking the patient to touch his or her nose and the examiner's finger in alternating fashion or running the heel down on the front of the shin. An important question which has to be answered: can the patient sit or even stand unaided? Is there compulsory lateropulsion out of proportion to the other complaints (central sign)? If no, gait and stance should be examined. Static posture may be tested by the Romberg test (ability to stand with the feet together and eyes closed). Patients with unilateral vestibular dysfunction veer (or fall) to the involved side, especially in the acute phase. Patients with bilateral vestibulopathy may perform well during this test, but usually fail on a thick foam carpet. The Unterberger (or Fukuda) stepping test and tandem walk challenge the vestibular system and cerebellar pathways.

5.2.3 Otological examination

Pathologies of the eardrum (acute or chronic otitis, eardrum perforation, herpetic bullae) should be noted. Rarely, it may be necessary to examine the eardrum using a microscope, since small perforations covered by a crust may hide the small openings of bigger cholesteatomas, of which the patient is unaware and which may grow expansively, destroying the SCCs or the facial nerve.

5.3 Instrumental examinations

5.3.1 Pure tone audiometry, acoustic reflex measurement

Pure tone audiometry (carried out to measure air- and bone-conduction) is an important, integral part of the neuro-otological examination battery. Even a bilaterally normal hearing threshold may aid diagnosis: in cases with BPPV, VN, and migrainous vertigo, hearing thresholds should or may be normal. In typical MD, unilateral low frequency hearing loss is an important clue, as is the the specific pattern of the loss: its fluctuations may contain some information about the involved side, stage, and severity. Slowly developing unilateral neural hearing loss may be caused by schwannoma of the cochleo-vestibular nerve. Sudden deafness in a patient with vascular risk factors and AVS may raise the possibility of stroke involving the AICA. Conductive hearing loss originating in the middle ear with short spontaneous vertigo spells may signal vertigo because of otosclerosis; conductive or combined hearing loss with vertigo which is provoked by sound or pressure (coughing, blowing nose) suggests SCC dehiscence. In these cases, a pathological additional window on the cochlea to the intracranial spaces created by the dehiscent superior canal results in dissipation of acoustic energy and is a cause of 'pseudo-conductive' hearing loss. Acoustic middle ear reflex (e.g. musculus stapedius) measurement is important in differentiating otosclerosis from dehiscence.

5.3.2 Evoked responses

The principle of evoked responses is based upon the averaging of event-related potentials elicited by short, repetitive stimuli. This method allows cancellation of noise and enhancement of a low intensity electrical signal. Previously, auditory brainstem response measurement (ABR) was used in cases with asymmetric sensorineural hearing loss to measure the conduction velocity of the cochlear nerve. This method made it possible to raise suspicion of vestibular schwannoma (VS) in 50% of the cases when the schwannoma was over 2cm. However, with the wide availability of magnetic resonance imaging (MRI), ABR has lost its significance as a screening method for tumours. In the meantime, the first wave of the ABR, the electrocochleographic potential complex has gained popularity in the clinical practice for measurement of endolymphatic hydrops. Having been widely used for measuring hearing function for decades, the technique of evoked responses using short, transient stimuli has recently also been introduced for the examination of vestibular reflexes.

5.3.3 Ecochg

By placing electrodes close to the inner ear, it is possible to record potentials evoked by the cochlear hair cells. The summating potential (SP) produced by the hair cells of the cochlea follows the envelope of the stimulus. It has been fairly well established in the literature that distension of the endolymphatic tube by experimental manipulations increases the amplitude of the SP (see also Section 6.3.3.2). Comparing SP amplitude values to the action potential (AP) amplitude, which usually does not decrease strongly in spite of the sensorineural hearing loss, it is possible to document displacement of the basilar membrane caused by increased endolymphatic pressure. Non-invasive electrode placement on the eardrum or even in the outer ear canal permits painless

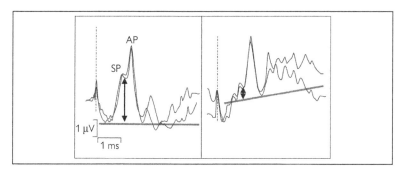

Figure 5.3 Click-evoked non-invasive Electrocochleographic potentials. Left panel: high SP/AP ratio in MD; right panel: normal curve. Every measurement was done twice in order to check reproducibility. SP and vertical arrows: summating potential; AP: action potential, vertical dotted line: time of the stimulus; horizontal grey line: baseline.

measurements which can be repeated to monitor changes or carried out on the other side to compare the two sides (see Figure 5.3).

Clinical significance. Although insufficient sensitivity, low specificity, and overlapping normal vs pathological values have been reported, many authors consider Ecochg to be important in the diagnosis and monitoring of MD. One of the present authors found it useful for verifying diagnosis before irreversible chemical ablation (Büki *et al* 2011) and noted even prognostic value in some cases.

5.3.4 Tests of otolithic function—ocular torsion and vestibular evoked myogenic potentials (VEMPs)

Subjective visuals—test of tonic otolithic function. Although normals can set a dimly lit bar within two degrees of the true gravitational horizontal or vertical even without visual cues, patients with unilateral vestibular lesions present with a roll-tilt of perceived vertical/horizontal. Shortly after an acute peripheral unilateral vestibular deafferentation (uVD), the deviation may reach up to 15 degrees towards the side of the lesion. It appears that the offset of the subjective visual horizontal (vertical) is due to tonic ocular torsion, one component of the OTR, which can be interpreted as the 'spontaneous nystagmus' of the otolithic system. With time it resolves almost completely; however, a slight offset may remain permanently. Offsets occur also in central otolithic dysfunction: patients with lower brainstem lesions involving the vestibular nucleus (e.g. lateral medullary infarctions) tilt the bar towards the side of the lesion, whereas upper brainstem lesions cause an offset away from the side of the lesion. Depending on the nuclei affected, cerebellar lesions may present with either contralesional or ipsilesional deviations (Baier *et al* 2008).

VEMP—a test of dynamic otolithic function. Since 1992, a new technique has been emerging for the examination of the vestibular periphery: VEMP testing (for review see Curthoys 2012). It is possible to stimulate the vestibular labyrinth by short duration air-conducted and bone-conducted vibrations. The stimuli activate otolithic receptors and initiate myogenic potentials in the effector muscles of the activated reflexes through sensitive irregular afferents. Air-conducted clicks and tone bursts applied through a

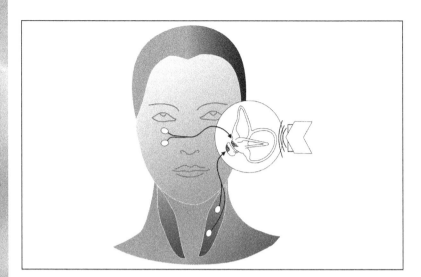

Figure 5.4 Principles of cVEMP and oVEMP examination.

headphone and bone-conducted vibrations stimulate both the utricle and the saccule. Since the saccule has strong neural connections to the ipsilateral sternocleidomastoid muscle, and the utricle projects strongly to the contralateral ocular muscles, by choosing the electrode montage to record myogenic electrical activity, it is possible to test the saccule (vestibulo-collic reflex arch) and the utricular VOR separately (Figure 5.4). Today, potentials evoked in the sternocleidomastoid muscle by air- or bone-conducted vibrations (cervical VEMP; cVEMP) are considered mainly as tests of ipsilateral saccular function and of the inferior vestibular nerve branch; myogenic potentials elicited in the inferior ocular muscles (ocular VEMP; oVEMP) are thought to be a test of the contralateral utricle and the superior branch of vestibular nerve.

When assessing the saccule and its nerve, the inferior branch, loud air-conducted clicks with intensities between 115 dB and 140 dB sound pressure or moderate bone-conducted vibrations may be used. The output is a short inhibitory-excitatory wave complex elicited in the ipsilateral sternocleidomastoid muscle via the cervical part of the vestibulo-spinal reflex arch. This so-called 'p13-n23 potential', named after direction and latency in milliseconds, appears if the muscle tension is sufficient with the head slightly elevated in supine position. The oVEMPs are recorded using two infraorbital electrodes. Using this electrode position, it is possible to minimize effects resulting from movements of the corneo-retinal dipole. If the patient is instructed to gaze upward, this places the belly of the inferior oblique muscle close to the electrode. In normals, bone-conducted vibrations applied on the forehead evoke symmetrical excitatory myogenic potentials (n10), probably mainly through the superior branch and contralateral utricular projections.

Clinical significance of otolithic tests. In VN, VEMPs supply information about the involved branches (superior, inferior, or both). In cases of isolated inferior branch involvement, cVEMPs may help to clarify the otherwise puzzling clinical picture of strong subjective vertigo without spontaneous nystagmus and with normal HIT. In superior canal dehiscence, oVEMP and cVEMP have enhanced amplitudes and reduced thresholds, because the third window on the labyrinth makes it susceptible to increased fluid movements due to vibrations.

References and Further Reading

Aw S. T., Haslwanter T., Fetter M. *et al.* (2000) Three-dimensional spatial characteristics of caloric nystagmus. *Exp Brain Res.* **134**, 289–94.

Baier B., Bense S., Dieterich M. (2008) Are signs of ocular tilt reaction in patients with cerebellar lesions mediated by the dentate nucleus? *Brain.* **131**, 1445–54.

Brodsky M. C., Donahue S. P., Vaphiades M. *et al.* (2006) Skew deviation revisited. *Surv Ophthalmol.* **51**, 105–28.

Büki B., Platz M., Haslwanter T. *et al.* (2011) Results of electrocochleography in Ménière's disease after successful vertigo control by single intratympanic gentamicin injection. *Audiol Neurootol.* **16**, 49–54.

Büttner U., Helmchen C., Brandt T. (1999) Diagnostic Criteria for Central versus Peripheral Positioning Nystagmus and Vertigo: a Review. *Acta Otolaryngol (Stockh).* **119**, 1–5.

Curthoys I. S. (2010) A critical review of the neurophysiological evidence underlying clinical vestibular testing using sound, vibration and galvanic stimuli. *Clin Neurophysiol.* **121**, 132–44.

Curthoys I. S. (2012) The interpretation of clinical tests of peripheral vestibular function. *Laryngoscope.* **122**, 1342–52.

Durrant J. D., Wang J., Ding D. L. *et al.* (1998) Are inner or outer hair cells the source of summating potentials recorded from the round window? *J Acoust Soc Am.* **104**, 370–7.

Ferraro J. A. and Durrant J D. (2006) Electrocochleography in the evaluation of patients with Ménière's disease/endolymphatic hydrops. *J Am Acad Audiol.* **17**, 45–68.

Halmagyi G. M. and Carey J. P. (2010) Vestibular evoked myogenic potentials—we live in interesting times. *Clin Neurophysiol.* **121**, 631–3.

Halmagyi G. M., Cremer P. D., Anderson J. *et al.* (2000) Isolated directional preponderance of caloric nystagmus: I. Clinical significance. *Am J Otol.* **21**, 559–67.

Lee H., Sohn S. I., Cho Y. W. *et al.* (2006) Cerebellar infarction presenting isolated vertigo: Frequency and vascular topographical patterns *Neurology.* **67**, 1178–83.

Leigh R. J. and Zee D. S. (eds). (2006) The neurology of eye movements. Oxford University Press.

Newman-Toker D. E., Sharma P., Chowdhury M. *et al.* (2009) Penlight-cover test: a new bedside method to unmask nystagmus. *J Neurol Neurosurg Psychiatry.* **80**, 900–3.

Rosengren S. M., Welgampola M. S., Colebatch J. G. (2010) Vestibular evoked myogenic potentials: past, present and future. *Clin Neurophysiol.* **121**, 636–51.

Salt A. N., Brown D. J., Hartsock J. J. *et al.* (2009) Displacements of the organ of Corti by gel injections into the cochlear apex. *Hear Res.* **250**, 63–75.

Tarnutzer A. A., Berkowitz A. L., Robinson K. A. *et al.* (2011) Does my dizzy patient have a stroke? A systematic review of bedside diagnosis in acute vestibular syndrome. *CMAJ.* **183**, E571–92.

Weber K. P., Aw S. T., Todd M. J. *et al.* (2008) Head impulse test in unilateral vestibular loss: vestibulo-ocular reflex and catch-up saccades. *Neurology.* **70**, 454–63.

Chapter 6

Three frequent peripheral causes of dizziness and vertigo

Key points
• Benign paroxysmal positional vertigo (BPPV) and Menière's disease (MD) are frequent diagnoses in specialized dizziness centres; vestibular neuritis is the most common peripheral cause of acute vestibular syndrome (AVS) in emergency settings.
• In BPPV, particles of the mass load of the linear accelerometer (utricular otoconia) escape and become mixed up with the mass load of the semicircular canals (SCCs) (endolymph), thereby sensitizing them to gravity and generating false information of angular acceleration after head position changes.
• The relative anatomical positions of the canals and the utricle explain all variants of peripheral paroxysmal positional nystagmus, the timing of the attacks, and the different frequencies by which the individual SCCs are affected.
• Analysis of nystagmus in provoking positions should be followed by reposition manoeuvres, which constitute effective bedside therapy methods.
• MD is characterized by fluctuating hearing loss, tinnitus, aural fullness and recurrent, spontaneous attacks of vertigo lasting up to two hours.
• Although MD is associated with endolymphatic hydrops, the primary pathogenic mechanism remains elusive.
• In MD, the progression of hearing loss cannot be stopped; but it is possible to control recurrent vertigo attacks by administering single intratympanic gentamicin injections.
• Vestibular neuritis (VN) is a frequent, benign, peripheral cause of isolated AVS.
• VN has three distinct patterns, corresponding to the three possible combinations of affected superior and inferior vestibular nerves (one or the other or both).

6.1 Introduction

Sudden, unilateral change of peripheral vestibular activity, either by decreasing or increasing afferent firing rate, causes asymmetry in the vestibular nuclei and corresponding modulation of vestibular signals (vestibulo-ocular, vestibulo-spinal reflexes, vegetative centres). Two of the three entities (BPPV and MD) discussed in this chapter cause recurrent complaints and are frequent diagnoses in specialized dizziness ambulances. The third, VN, is the most common peripheral cause of AVS, with dizziness lasting more than 24 hours, encountered usually in emergency settings.

6.2 BPPV

The peripheral vestibular organ consists of miniature inertial accelerometers: the SCCs, specialized in angular velocity changes and the otolithic organs measuring linear accelerations, including gravity. Generally, accelerometers have the following components: mass load, on which acceleration forces act; the sensor, which is sensitive to the movements of the mass; and a damped spring, which connects the two (Table 6.1).

In BPPV, according to the accepted theory, particles of the mass load of the linear accelerometer (utricular otoconial debris) escape and become mixed up with the mass load of the SCCs (endolymph), thereby sensitizing them to gravity and generating false information on angular acceleration. Once in the SCC, debris gravitates always to the most inferior part of the canal. Head position changes cause movements of the debris inducing pathological endolymph flow with a certain latency, which in turn conveys the false perception of acceleration. Current models of BPPV incorporate only utricular otoconia, because the utriculus and the SCC ampullae share the same fluid compartment, in contrast to the sacculus, which is only connected to the utricle by a thin channel, the utriculo-saccular duct. Although we shall see that saccular otoconia are apt to degenerate even earlier during life than utricular ones, there have been no theories put forward to explain symptoms (whichever symptoms these might be) caused by dislodged saccular otoconia (Figure 6.1).

In BPPV, all symptoms and signs (nystagmus) can be explained by considering possible movements of dislodged utricular otoconial debris in the three-dimensional structure of the vestibular labyrinth.

6.2.1 Otoconia formation and maintenance

In mammals, otoconia formation occurs during embryonic life and, in contrast to the single otolith of the teleost fish, which continues to grow indefinitely, there is most probably only a slow turnover of the otoconia material, calcium carbonate, during adult life. Endolymph calcium concentration in the utriculus is one tenth of that of the plasma (0.25 mM and 2.6 mM respectively); therefore, in order for $CaCO_3$ to crystallize, otoconia organic components must be able to actively sequester Ca^{2+} so as to efficiently raise its microenvironmental concentration. The calcification of otoconia is a tightly regulated process (for review see Lundberg et al 2006) starting with the seeding of crystals by the sequestration of Ca^{2+} by a protein, otoconin 90 (Oc90), to form $Oc90-CaCO_3$, which then recruits other minor proteins. These

Table 6.1 Elements of the vestibular accelerometers

	Otolithic organs	SCCs
Mass	Otoconia	Endolymph
Spring	Damped viscoelastic gelatinous matrix of the macular sensory epithelium	Damped viscoelastic gelatinous matrix of the cupulae
Sensor	Vestibular hair cells of the utricular and saccular maculae	Vestibular hair cells of the cupulae of the SCCs
Movements of the mass	Shearing movement in the plane of the (curved) macular surface in any direction due to tangential linear acceleration	Inertial movement of the endolymph fluid during angular acceleration of the head, only in the plane of the canal

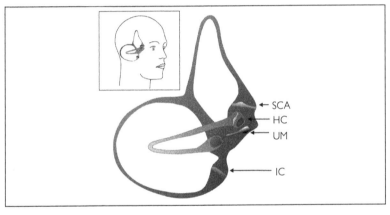

Figure 6.1 Explanation of sketches used in this chapter. UM: Utricular macula; SC: superior canal ampulla; HC: horizontal canal ampulla; IC: inferior (posterior) canal ampulla. The caudal part of the utricular macula is floating on a thin membrane (Uzun-Coruhlu et al 2007).

free-floating, minute Oc90-$CaCO_3$ seeds may be seen in the endolymph even at a distance away from the macula region. As a second stage of otoconia formation, a slightly acidic microenvironmental pH near the stereocilia of the macular hair cells attracts otoconial proteins and at the same time prevents accretion of $CaCO_3$ too close to the hair bundles (acidic pH increases solubility of calcium carbonate, alkaline pH acts opposite, conserving otoconia). Extrusion of Ca^{2+} and HCO_3^- from hair cells and secretion of other proteins from the macula are critical for on-site growth and possibly maintenance of otoconia. The otoconia crystals (Figure 6.2), which have an organic central core and mineral peripheral zones, are partially embedded in a membranous/fibrous matrix and are anchored by protein filaments to the kinocilium of the underlying hair cells.

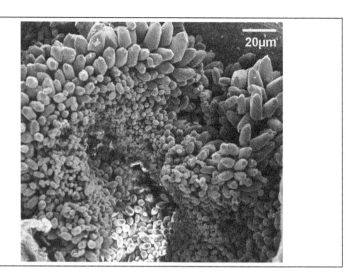

Figure 6.2 Otoconia of the mouse (Photo by courtesy of Yunxia W. Lundberg, Vestibular Neurogenetics Laboratory, Boys Town National Research Hospital, Omaha, Nebraska, USA)

6.2.2 Pathophysiology of BPPV

It is likely that changes in this finely tuned ionic microenvironment and fragility of anchoring protein filaments could be brought about by ageing, eliciting otoconial degeneration and dislocation. Using scanning electron microscopy, signs of age-related changes were demonstrated in several studies (for review see Thalmann et al 2001). Surface pitting, hollowing out, fragmentation, and dislodgement of saccular otoconia starting at about age 50–60 years is usually followed by similar changes in the utriculus (Ross et al 1976). Since Ca^{2+} extruded by vestibular hair cells maintains otoconial substance, it is tempting to speculate that otoconial degeneration in the elderly is connected to the age-dependent decline in the vestibular hair cell counts: in pathological studies of the group of Dr Merchant (Massachusetts Eye and Ear Infirmary), there was a highly significant age-related decline in all sense organs for total, type I, and type II hair cell densities, which was best fit by a linear regression model (Merchant et al 2000). BPPV may occur after head trauma; it is possible that in these cases relatively healthy otoconia are dislodged because of rupturing anchor proteins. Association with VN may show the pathophysiological significance of ionic and metabolic changes caused by disturbances of microcirculation: following an attack of VN, many patients develop posterior canal type BPPV on the affected side and, conversely, previous VN can be found frequently in the history of patients with BPPV. In this special constellation, the neuritis involves the upper part of the end-organ, including the utriculus but sparing the posterior ampulla, which may thus relay pathological information caused by displaced otoconial debris.

The course of BPPV is often benign—dislodged otoconia may perhaps be dissolved—however, sometimes symptoms may persist for months, suggesting that, under

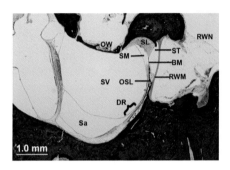

Figure 3.5 Histological section through the labyrinth showing the relation of stapes movements to the saccular macula. The close relationship between the stapes footplate (here seen in the oval window (OW)) makes the sacculus (Sa) and the utricular macula (running vertically, left from the sacculus) especially sensitive to sound. BM: Organ of Corti on the basilar membrane; RWM: round window membrane; OSL: osseous spiral lamina; SV: scala vestibuli; ST: scala tympani; RWN: round window niche; DR: ductus reuniens; SL: spiral ligament. Reprinted with permission from Li PM, Wang H, Northrop C, Merchant SN, Nadol JB Jr. Anatomy of the round window and hook region of the cochlea with implications for cochlear implantation and other endocochlear surgical procedures. Otol Neurotol. 2007 Aug;28(5):641–8. © Wolters Kluwer Health, 2007.

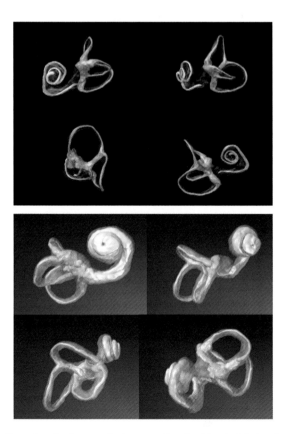

Figure 6.11 Three-dimensional computerized reconstruction of endolymphatic hydrops from specimens of temporal bone. Upper panel: normal controls; views from four different directions (yellow: endolymphatic space in the cochlea). Lower panels: Specimen with hydrops (yellow). The authors digitalized sections of temporal bone and reconstructed the inner ear spaces in three dimensions. Reproduced by permission from Teranishi *et al* (2009), © Taylor and Francis (2007).

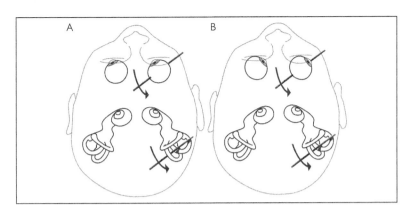

Figure 6.3 Activation of SCCs. Axis of eye rotation is approximately parallel and fixed to the sensitivity vector of the affected SCC. The movements of the pupils, however, depend on the gaze direction: A. With a gaze to the left, the ensuing nystagmus is vertical. B. With a gaze to the right, the ensuing nystagmus is purely rotatory.

pathologic conditions (e.g. perhaps in osteoporosis or osteopenia, Vibert *et al* 2003), this process may be slowed down.

Involvement of different SCCs. Otoconial debris may affect all three SCCs. In three-dimensional space, the axis of eye rotation is approximately parallel to the sensitivity vector of the affected SCC, independent of gaze position. That means, on the other hand, that the apparent movements of the pupils seem to change with gaze position. With the involvement of the right posterior SCC, for example, the pupils move mainly vertically during gaze to the left; with gaze to the right however, rotational nystagmus components dominate. (Figure 6.3).

Mechanism of canalolithiasis. In a supine position, the common crus of the vertical SCC opens immediately below the utricular macula (Figure 6.4). The horizontal canal opening is also below the utriculus; however, it is directed laterally. It is easy to speculate that, in supine position (during a night's rest), debris may fall into the vertical canals. During sitting up, the fate of the debris is different in the individual canals. By raising the head, the patient may involuntarily liberate the superior SCC (eliciting subjective vertigo and vegetative complaints). This hypothetical mechanism may explain the rarity of the superior canal canalolithiasis. In contrast, otoconial granules in the posterior SCC move further in the direction of the cupula and become trapped in the most inferior region of the SCC, which is closed by the cupula on the other, utricular side. Then, it is only possible to remove the debris from the posterior canal by a 'backward somersault'. Consequently, the Epley manoeuvre is basically a backward somersault carried out with a U-turn (see Section 6.2.6.1).

Sometimes free-floating debris enters the horizontal canal. Here too, spontaneous recovery may occur when patients turn over in bed. The relative geometrical arrangement of the utriculus and SCCs may explain the timing of the attacks (usually in the morning) and the different frequencies by which the individual SCCs are affected (see Section 6.2.4). Symptoms caused by lateral canalolithiasis may start seemingly

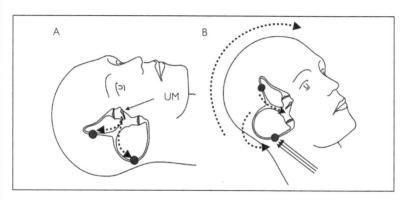

Figure 6.4 Relative position of the vertical SCCs and the utricular macula in the supine position. A. In supine position (during sleep), the opening of the vertical canals is below the macula. B. During sitting up, the superior canal may be inadvertently freed from debris; otoconial mass in the poste-rior canal becomes trapped in the most inferior part of the canal (triple arrow). UM: utricular macula.

spontaneously any time during the day, evoked by slight, sideways head movements in the roll plane.

6.2.3 Epidemiology

Although BPPV is undoubtedly the most common diagnosis in patients visiting dizziness outpatients departments, its incidence in the overall population is not known because most studies aimed to determine this value had methodological limitations (either carried out on the telephone, or examining only patients seeking help with acute symptoms). A study with particularly impressive results showed the importance of ageing: 9% of a public, inner-city geriatric population had unrecognized BPPV (Oghalai et al 2000). These patients were more likely to have reduced activities and to have sustained a fall in the previous three months.

6.2.4 Symptoms

BPPV usually starts during the night, when the patient is turning over in bed, or in the morning, when sitting up for the first time during or after the night's rest. This first attack may be threatening and strong enough to cause a disability for one or two days, although, when lying completely motionless, patients do not experience strong vertigo. Patients may be able to walk, albeit feeling dizzy. During hours or days, debris conglomerates may be dispersed, or SCCs may be spontaneously liberated by movements; and eventually the strongest symptoms disappear. However, short vertigo spells during head movements (when looking up, bending forward, or turning over in bed) may persist for a longer time.

6.2.5 Examination

Diagnosis of BPPV requires the detection of positioning or positional nystagmus provoked by Dix-Hallpike (for vertical SCC) or supine roll (for horizontal SCC) manoeuvres, which indicates canalo- or cupolithiasis of the affected SCC.

Dix-Hallpike position consists of initially turning the patient's head by 45 degrees in yaw toward the side to be examined, and then pitching the patient backwards by 130 degrees from upright, to ear-down, head-hanging position, i.e. approximately 40 degrees below earth-horizontal (Aw et al 2005). Horizontal supine roll can be carried out in supine position by turning the head of the patient 90 degrees right and left in the corresponding lateral positions. Although the magnitude of the nystagmus is somewhat reduced with visual fixation, it is usually easily seen without efforts by the examiner to reduce fixation (examination in the dark or under Frenzel's goggles is not absolutely necessary in a routine clinical setting).

Nomenclature. Since in Dix-Hallpike position the patient's head is hanging upside down, an upbeat nystagmus with a fast component toward the centre of the earth also beats towards the top of the head; therefore, it is called upbeat geotropic. Conversely, nystagmus beating down, in the direction of the chin, is called positional downbeat nystagmus; however in head-hanging position, this is in fact apogeotropic. The torsional component is named by the fast movement of the upper pole of the eyes.

Canalolithiasis-cupulolithiasis. Dislodged debris may move freely in the SCCs (canalolithiasis) or adhere to the cupulae and deflect them in different head positions (cupulolithiasis). In this latter case, the nystagmus (and the symptoms) may be less intense and may last longer. In case of the horizontal canal, nystagmus occurs in opposite directions in **canalo-** versus **cupulo**lithiasis after sideways head roll in supine position. This is because otoconial precipitates in the horizontal canal move opposite to the direction of the gravity induced paradoxical cupular deflection (Section 6.2.6.2).

Concerning the anterior canals, the Dix-Hallpike position should theoretically elicit the movements of debris in the same direction in both canalo- and cupulolithiasis.

This is not so straightforward in the posterior canals. In posterior canal **canalo**lithiasis, when the patient is positioned from sitting into a head-hanging position, the debris moves away from the utriculus in the posterior canal (Section 6.2.6.1). In posterior **cupulo**lithiasis, in an upright position, the debris adhering to the posterior cupula (perhaps after being deposited on it from above) deflects it downwards, away from the utriculus. Then, depending on the exact anatomical angle of the ampulla (this varies, Bradshaw 2010) and on the actual angle of the hanging-head position, either nothing changes in Dix-Hallpike position (therefore no nystagmus ensues (Figure 6.5A, D)) or, in the case of a more inferiorly attached ampulla, the cupula deflects upward towards the utriculus in Dix-Hallpike position, causing a slight, prolonged downbeat nystagmus, which could be indistinguishable from an anterior (superior) canalolithiasis (Figure 6.5B, C). Such a downbeat nystagmus could hypothetically be elicited bilaterally, from both Dix-Hallpike positions and also in straight head-hanging position (note, peripheral downbeat nystagmus elicited by posterior canal cupulolithiasis is predicted to be prolonged in duration, exceeding the usual duration of canalolithiasis (5–20 seconds), possibly allowing a distinction from peripheral downbeat nystagmus in anterior canal canalolithiasis). Although the three-dimensional reconstructions in Figure 6.11 were not done by Teranishi et al (2009) with the intention to demonstrate the angle of insertion of the inferior ampulla into the vestibulum, it is clearly to be seen that, in the control specimen, this happens from a rather inferior position. Apparently, the inferior ampulla (and therefore, as a diaphragm, the cupula containing the hair cells) is the most inferior part of the endolymphatic space, which also contains the utricular macula, housing thousands of otoconia. This should be

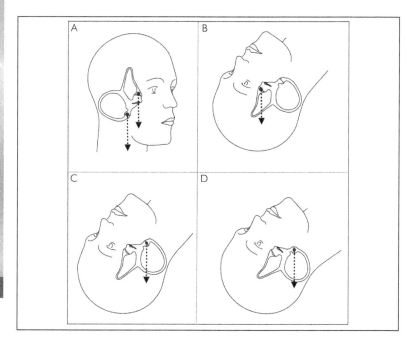

Figure 6.5 Hypothetical mechanisms of peripheral downbeat nystagmus in BPPV. A. Anterior and posterior cupulolithiasis in sitting (vertical arrows, effects of gravity). B. Anterior cupulolithiasis in Dix-Hallpike position. C. Posterior cupulolithiasis; in a case of perhaps more inferiorly connecting ampulla and more pronounced head-hanging position, the cupula may be deflected toward the utriculus, thereby eliciting a slight downbeat nystagmus. D. In a case of an anatomically less inferior connecting ampulla and in a less pronounced Dix-Hallpike position, the cupula, which is already deflected in sitting, does not change its position during the provocative manoeuvre; no nystagmus ensues.

taken into account when thinking about BPPV (see also the cartoon by Schuknecht in Figure 12.2).

6.2.6 BPPV canal types and their therapy

Cases with canalolithiasis can and should be solved by repositioning or liberation manoeuvres. It is easy to speculate that, in cupulolithiasis, it may be difficult to offer an immediate solution; however, there is usually no need for therapy, because symptoms are mild and resolve spontaneously. In their carefully designed study, Aw *et al* (2005) examined cases with BPPV using the magnetic scleral search coil technique. This method allowed the authors to document the eye movements in different BPPV variants very exactly. By comparing nystagmus rotation axes to SCC axes, the authors could identify affected canals (Table 6.2).

6.2.6.1 *Posterior (inferior) canalolithiasis*

In this (most frequent) variant, in response to the Dix–Hallpike test, the nystagmus is upbeat geotropic-torsional toward the lowermost ear. The time course is paroxysmal,

Table 6.2 Nystagmus* in different types of BPPV

	Canalolithiasis	Cupulolithiasis
Posterior Canal	Geotropic-torsional upbeat nystagmus with short latency, provoked when the affected ear is lowermost in the Dix–Hallpike position	Depending on anatomy, either no nystagmus after positioning the patient from sitting into Dix–Hallpike position, or sometimes possibly downbeat
Horizontal Canal	Geotropic horizontal (beating laterally down in both lateral supine positions)	Apogeotropic horizontal (beating laterally up in both lateral supine positions)
Superior Canal	Apogeotropic downbeat nystagmus with a small torsional fast phase which beats toward the affected ear; possible to elicit by Dix-Hallpike test to either side	Same as in superior canalolithiasis (apogeotropic downbeat) but beginning almost immediately; less paroxysmal and more persistent

* Nystagmus provoked by positioning the patient into the Dix-Hallpike position from sitting (vertical canals affected) or by rolling the head sideways from the supine position (horizontal canal affected) (Aw et al 2005).

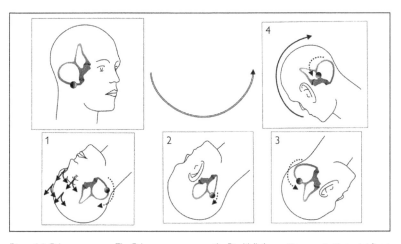

Figure 6.6 Epley manoeuvre. The Epley manoeuvre uses the Dix-Hallpike position as a starting point (inset 1). This can be considered as the first part of a backward somersault. Then the patient's head is turned toward the other side by 180 degrees to a nose-down position (inset 2-3); then the second part of the backward rotation can be carried out when the head is elevated (inset 4).

with a latency of several seconds and a duration of 5–20 seconds. For therapy, several manoeuvres have been designed. A slow and therefore gentle way of moving the otoconial debris away from the closed end of the canal toward the opening and into the vestibule has been proposed by Epley (1992) (Figure 6.6). During the manoeuvre, the patients experience vertigo, and continual upbeat nystagmus can be observed as the debris travels along the SCC. The manoeuver can be repeated several times until no nystagmus and vertigo can be evoked. In some cases, after a successful Epley manoeuvre, simultaneous canalolithiasis of the horizontal canal can be unmasked, or the iatrogenic shift of the debris in another canal (superior or horizontal) can be observed. In these cases, perhaps with intermissions in order not to produce a strong, vegetative reaction, successive repositions are indicated.

6.2.6.2 Horizontal canalo- and cupulolithiasis

In canalolithiasis, in response to a supine roll test, the nystagmus is bilaterally horizontal geotropic in the lateral supine position, being more intense on the affected side (Figure 6.7). Search coil measurements demonstrate a minimal torsional component, which is mostly missed by visual observation. The nystagmus is paroxysmal, with a few seconds latency, and may be very intense, causing a strong vegetative reaction.

In cupulolithiasis, the nystagmus is bilaterally apogeotropic, with an almost invisible, small apogeotropic-torsional component. It shows a flattened, longer velocity profile. It is usually less intense and has longer duration, although in some acute cases it may be surprisingly intensive. It is stronger with the affected ear uppermost because endolymph flow towards the cupula causes a more intensive reaction than a movement away from it.

Therapy for horizontal canalolithiasis consists of a barbecue roll toward the contralateral side (Figure 6.8). Before the roll, short to-and-fro movements may be necessary in order to disperse the debris. In spite of correct repositioning, horizontal canalolithiasis may be persistent, probably because the otoconial fragments get stuck before the opening or because they fall out but then immediately return into the SCC opening during the rotation. It may require repeated manoeuvres (with pauses, because of the vegetative reaction), sometimes even over several days. The vegetative reaction may be reduced by the administration of antihistaminic vestibular suppressants before repeated reposition.

In horizontal cupulolithiasis, the patient should carry out repeated head shaking or barbecue rolls.

In acute BPPV of the horizontal canals, sometimes the so-called 'lying-down nystagmus' may be elicited when the patient reclines from sitting to supine position. In an emergency situation, this transient phenomenon may be mistaken for a spontaneous nystagmus. It has been suggested that it is caused by gravity-dependent movements of the otolithic debris in the horizontal canal.

6.2.6.3 Anterior canalo- and cupulolithiasis

Nystagmus for anterior canalo- and cupulolithiasis is predominantly downbeat, with only a small torsional component. The torsional fast phase of the nystagmus beats toward the affected ear but is very small and may easily be missed on visual observation. In the Dix-Hallpike position, the ipsilateral inferior and contralateral superior canals are in the plane of the positioning (see left anterior right posterior (LARP) and right anterior left posterior (RALP) planes; Chapter 3). So, in principle, nystagmus in anterior canalo/cupulolithiasis should only be provoked in the Dix-Hallpike position contralateral to the affected ear. However, Aw *et al* (2005) showed that

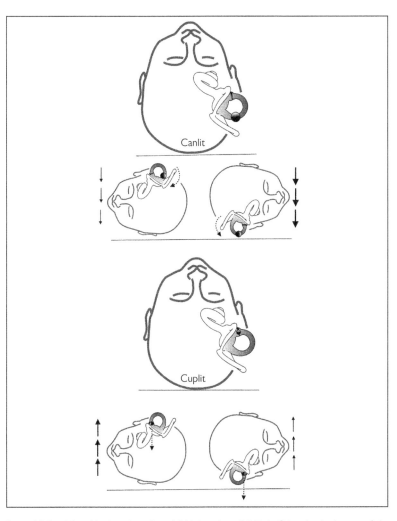

Figure 6.7 Principles of horizontal canal canalolithiasis and cupulolithiasis. Other than in the case of the vertical canals, debris moves differently in horizontal canalolithiasis (Canlit) and cupulolithiasis (Cuplit) after assuming the provoking (lateral supine) position. Upper panels (Canlit): In both lateral positions, movements of the debris cause geotropic horizontal nystagmus (arrows) which is stronger on the affected side. Lower panels (Cuplit): in cupulolithiasis, slight and protracted apogeotropic nystagmus ensues in both lateral positions and is somewhat stronger with the affected ear upper-most.

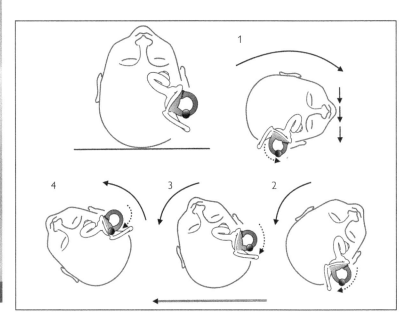

Figure 6.8 Barbecue roll to solve a right canalolithiasis. Inset 1: Right lateral position. When the geotropic nystagmus disappears, a slow rotation to the left moves the particles along the canal (insets 2-4).

it is possible to elicit nystagmus bilaterally. This phenomenon is possibly because of the anatomy: the superior SCC ampulla is above the posterior SCC ampulla; otoconia in the superior SCC ampulla would still be able to gravitate toward the superior SCC limb in a Dix-Hallpike test to the affected ear. The special anatomical position of this canal also explains why it is not necessary to devise a repositioning manoeuvre for this canal: once in Dix-Hallpike position, it is only necessary to bring the patient again into an upright, sitting position. If this is carried out slowly, reposition automatically occurs (see Figure 6.4). Also, this is why this variant may be extremely rare. In other canal variants, especially upbeat geotropic nystagmus in inferior (posterior) canalolithiasis, peripheral lithiasis is much more frequent than are central causes. Peripheral downbeat nystagmus in Dix-Hallpike position may also possibly be elicited by an acute dislocation of otoconia from the utricular macula directly onto the superior ampulla (which lies immediately below the macula in the Dix-Hallpike position); or by posterior cupulolithiasis. Although, according to new data, peripheral downbeat nystagmus due to BPPV may be more frequent than supposed so far (Chapter 12), one should always bear in mind that central positional downbeat nystagmus is common and may also be elicited by potentially dangerous pathologies (such as cerebellar or spinocerebellar degeneration, multiple sclerosis (MS), Arnold-Chiari malformation, lithium toxicity, paraneoplastic disease, and primary cerebellar tumour).

6.2.6.4 Combined inferior (posterior) and horizontal canalolithiasis

Sometimes an oblique nystagmus may be provoked (i.e. mixed geotropic horizontal and upbeating) with a disproportionately large geotropic-torsional component toward the lowermost ear either in the Dix-Hallpike or supine ear-down test. Aw *et al* (2005) explained this observation by combined canalolithiasis of the posterior and horizontal canals. In these cases, the Epley manoeuvre unmasks the horizontal component, which then can be solved by the corresponding sequential barbecue roll.

6.2.6.5 Subjective BPPV

Neurotologists regularly see patients with typical complaints of BPPV (short vertigo when bending forward, lying down, sitting up, or turning over in bed), but without provoked nystagmus, even with repeated provocation manoeuvres. In has been suggested that this 'subjective' BPPV may be more frequent than previously thought; (for a hypothetical explanation and possible therapeutic manoeuvres, see Chapter 12).

6.2.7 Differential diagnosis

In the case of typical symptoms and transient geotropic nystagmus upon Dix-Hallpike provocation that then cannot be elicited after an Epley manoeuvre (such as with inferior canalolithiasis), the examiner may be confident about the correct diagnosis. However, in all other cases there may be some doubt about a possible central cause. In their review, Büttner *et al* (1999) stated that it is not possible to differentiate between peripheral BPPV and positionally triggered central nystagmus according to latency, horizontal direction of nystagmus, fatigability, and the crescendo–decrescendo type of nystagmus during an attack. Central origin has to be assumed for purely upbeat, down-beat, and pure torsional nystagmus. In particular, downbeat nystagmus should alert the examiner to a possible central pathology, although it may be caused by peripheral lithiasis (see Section 6.2.6.3). A slight peripheral spontaneous nystagmus may also be confused with a positional one if it is missed during examination in sitting posture, since it may be amplified in Dix-Hallpike or lateral supine position. From a practical point, it is recommended to search for a central cause of positional vertigo (including using brain magnetic resonance imaging (MRI)), especially if either the pattern of nystagmus does not fit one of the typical BPPV types or if treatment for BPPV is insufficient (Figure 6.9).

6.2.8 Prognosis

Although some BPPV cases are benign and resolve even spontaneously, recurrence is common. In a recent study, the recurrence rate of BPPV was 27%, and relapse largely occurred in the first six months (Perez *et al* 2012). At present, the generally accepted recurrence rate of BPPV after successful treatment is 40–50% at five years of average follow-up. A subset of individuals appears prone to multiple recurrences. There are new data concerning this group of patients. Although connections between vitamin D deficiency and osteoporosis, as well as between osteoporosis and BPPV, have been suggested in the literature, a possible link between vitamin D and BPPV has been suggested only recently. Büki *et al* (2012) proposed that patients with recurrent BPPV might benefit from vitamin D supplementation if their serum 25-OH-vitamin D levels

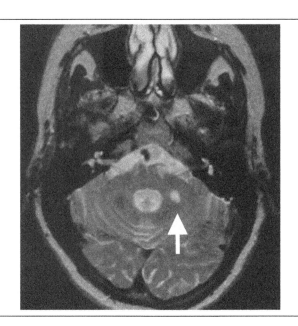

Figure 6.9 MRI image of a small cerebellar infarction (arrow) causing geotropic horizontal positional nystagmus in a lateral supine position

were low. Jeong *et al* (2012) also found a statistical association between idiopathic BPPV and decreased serum vitamin D. Further statistical epidemiological investigations will help to determine if there is a beneficial effect of correcting vitamin D deficiency on the recurrence of BPPV. Even until these results are available, given the other known benefits of vitamin D, measurement and, if necessary, supplementation with vitamin D may be useful.

6.3 **Menière's disease (MD)**

MD is characterized by spontaneous attacks of vertigo/dizziness, fluctuating sensorineural hearing loss, sensation of aural fullness, and tinnitus. It has an estimated prevalence (number of cases present in a given population at a certain time) of between 15 and 500 per 100,000 inhabitants. MD is a clinically significant entity because it may have serious consequences for the affected persons, when constantly recurring, unanticipated attacks make normal life and—in some occupations—the professional career of the patient impossible. Nowadays, the fluctuating, paradoxical activity of the affected vestibular organ can be gently inhibited, thereby preventing the recurrence of vertigo attacks. However, the progression of hearing loss cannot be halted.

6.3.1 Pathophysiology of MD

Already more than 70 years ago it had been suggested (Hallpike and Cairns 1938; Yamakawa 1938) and today is universally accepted that an increase of the endolymphatic volume (endolymphatic hydrops) is associated with MD (Figures 6.10 and 6.11). The hydrops may be considered secondary in cases with prior surgical trauma, temporal bone fracture, labyrinthitis, chronic otitis, otosyphilis, Cogan's syndrome, and even

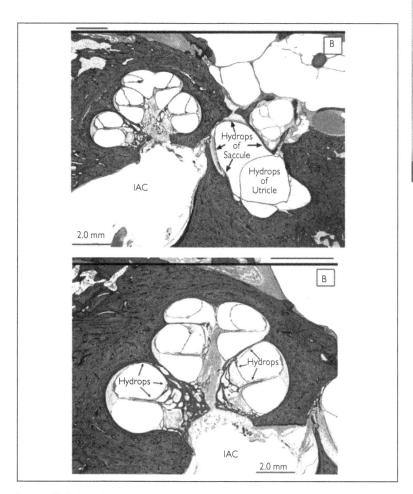

Figure 6.10 Cochlear histopathology in MD. Reproduced with permission from Chung *et al* (2011), © Wolters Kluwer Health, 2011.

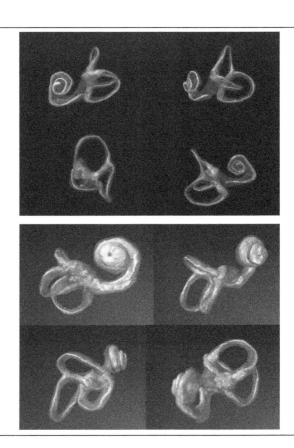

Figure 6.11 Three-dimensional computerized reconstruction of endolymphatic hydrops from specimens of temporal bone. Upper panel: normal controls; views from four different directions (yellow: endolymphatic space in the cochlea). Lower panels: Specimen with hydrops (yellow). The authors digitalized sections of temporal bone and reconstructed the inner ear spaces in three dimensions. Reproduced by permission from Teranishi *et al* (2009), © Taylor and Francis (2007). See also colour plate section.

(possibly viral induced) earlier sudden hearing loss. However, in the majority of MD cases, no possible cause can be found. It is even uncertain if hydrops is a link in the pathophysiologic chains of events. In a recent histopathologic study, Merchant *et al* (2005) stated that, although in all cases with MD, endolymphatic hydrops can be seen upon histopathological examination, hydrops of the cochlea and/or vestibular system is not necessarily associated with a history of episodic vertigo. The authors found cases with histologic endolymphatic hydrops and sensorineural hearing loss but without a history of vertigo. One is tempted to accept their reasoning that the results were not consistent with the 'central hypothesis of hydrops as the final common pathway for production of symptoms' in MD. The authors remark that hydrops may be a marker for disordered homeostasis of the labyrinth, in which an unknown factor produces both the clinical symptoms of MD and endolymphatic hydrops.

In addition, the mechanism of an actual attack is unknown. Schuknecht (1963) suggested that, with rupture of distended membranes, high K^+-concentration endolymph mixes with perilymph and floods hair cell bodies and nerve endings; it has been also observed that Ca^{++}-concentration of the endolymph increases in animal models of hydrops (for a review see Salt and Plontke 2010). Both ionic imbalances would temporarily inhibit tonic spontaneous peripheral vestibular firing. However, Rabbitt et al (2001) showed that subtle changes in endolymph pressure might per se modulate SCC primary afferent discharge. Thus, transient pressure waves could also elicit paradoxical activity changes (and attacks) without ruptures of the membrane containing endolymph.

6.3.2 Symptoms

Because patients with MD usually do not have attacks at the time of examination, diagnosis often relies on the anamnestic presentation of typical symptoms: feelings of pressure or fullness in the affected ear, sudden and spontaneous vertigo spells (with vegetative symptoms) preceded or accompanied by episodes of hearing loss, and loud tinnitus. The attacks last for minutes or longer, maximally for 2–3 hours. In earlier stages, low frequency hearing loss is typical, and hearing may recover between attacks. With such a typical presentation, it is not difficult to make the diagnosis. Later, during the course of the disease, however, permanent sensorineural hearing loss develops. Also, there exists another typical course: sudden unilateral hearing loss, which does not recover, with vertigo attacks manifesting years later (this may be called 'delayed hydrops'). In cases in which permanent hearing loss has already developed, patients may not notice anything such as louder tinnitus, fluctuating hearing, or transient hearing loss in the affected ear during or preceding the attack. In other rare cases, several monosymptomatic vertigo attacks occur, and hearing loss develops later. In both of the latter groups, the diagnosis may be difficult.

Lermoyez syndrome. Sometimes, usually in the early stages, hearing loss and the sensation of fullness in the ear become more and more troubling over days; and then these symptoms suddenly improve during a vertigo attack. This is called the Lermoyez variant. Another troubling symptom, which occurs in approximately 6% of all MD cases, is Tumarkin's drop attack ('otolithic crisis'). Drop attacks consist of sudden loss of muscular tonus and fall or collapse of the patient with intact consciousness. Patients may sustain traumatic injuries because they cannot support themselves during the fall. Luckily, as we shall see, intratympanic gentamicin therapy also inhibits the Tumarkin attacks, which may possibly develop because of paroxysmal pathological activity of saccular afferents.

6.3.3 Diagnostic methods

In 2004, Minor et al stated in a review that 'there is no single feature or subset of features from the history, physical examination, or diagnostic tests that establishes the diagnosis of Menière's disease with certainty.' The situation has not changed since. In the early course of the disease, there are no symptoms and signs between attacks; therefore, between attacks, bedside and instrumental test give normal results. In cases with progression, slowly permanent defects develop; then it is possible to demonstrate some characteristic patterns of audio-vestibular hypofunction. However, most of the single test results are only pathologic in a certain percentage of the cases and can be used only in the context with other results. Apart from the history of complaints, the most useful diagnostic data come from testing cochlear function. The diagnostic difficulties and uncertainties are mirrored in the guidelines set up by the American Academy of Otolaryngology—Head and Neck Surgery (Monsell *et al* 1995). Here the criteria of 'definite MD' are two or more spontaneous episodes of vertigo, each lasting 20 minutes or longer, hearing loss documented by audiograms on at least one occasion (even if it is not fluctuating), and tinnitus or aural fullness in the affected ear, other causes excluded.

6.3.3.1 Bedside tests

On the rare occasions when the doctor is present during an attack, the documentation of the spontaneous nystagmus may deliver diagnostic information. Sometimes the initial nystagmus is irritative, i.e. beating towards the ear with feeling of pressure and fluctuating hearing with the head impulse test (HIT) being normal bilaterally. Then, a spontaneous nystagmus follows as a result of the transient loss of vestibular activity on the affected side, with the fast phase beating towards the contralateral side. During this second phase, the vestibular loss can be demonstrated by the HIT, which is positive toward the affected side. Then, a recovery nystagmus ensues, beating again towards the ipsilateral side, with again a normal HIT bilaterally. Although the course of an attack is not always typical, when these phases can be documented, it has diagnostic significance; hence the observation of nystagmus (preventing fixation by Frenzel's goggles or other techniques) in the emergency setting may be important.

Sometimes a positive Hennebert's sign can be found in ears with MD: positive or negative pressure applied in the outer ear canal causes (mostly horizontal) eye movements and dizziness (possibly because a distended endolymphatic membrane contacts the stapes footplate).

6.3.3.2 Tests of cochlear function

Pure tone audiometry. In the early stages, fluctuating low frequency hearing loss associated with the vertigo attack is an important clue, sometimes with a slight air-bone gap (for which again the saccule may be responsible by touching the stapes footplate, increasing stiffness and changing the impedance of the stapes vibrations, see upper panel of Figure 6.10). In the course of the disease, over years, with the development of a more pronounced, permanent, unilateral hearing loss, pure tone threshold is usually flat (Savastano *et al* 2006). In a study of Büki *et al* (2012), threshold around 2000–3000 Hz was significantly better than around 250–500–750 Hz in a group of 62 patients with **advanced** MD and flat audiogram. In Figure 6.12, we show our own unpublished results of 94 patients with MD (including the data of the 62 patients analysed in Büki *et al* 2012). This group was homogenous because all patients had severe complaints, frequent attacks, and needed/accepted intratympanic gentamicin therapy. The audiograms in this group show a rather homogenous flat pattern in spite of the big number of cases; again the small but highly significant upward 'bump' at 2 kHz can be seen.

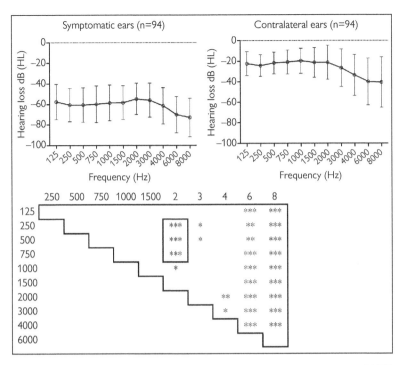

Figure 6.12 Typical flat hearing loss in advanced MD (average + SD). Lower panel: one way ANOVA (Friedman test) and the results of Dunn's multiple comparison post test of the different frequency bands shown in the upper left panel (symptomatic ear). Every frequency was compared to every other frequency on the same side; *p < 0.05; **p < 0.01; ***p < 0.001. When p > 0.05 (no significant difference), the crossing point was left empty. High frequencies differ significantly from lower or middle frequencies; in addition, on the symptomatic side, the difference between the hearing threshold at 2 kHz and that at 250, 500, and 750 Hz is highly significant (box).

Electrocochleography (Ecochg; see also Chapter 5.3.3). An electrode placed close to the cochlea records the electrical activity of cochlear hair cells. One of the potentials recorded by the electrode is a direct current, a steady change following the envelope of the stimulus, called the summating potential (SP). The SP results mainly from the transduction process of the inner hair cells. During transduction, stimulus vibrations are translated into electrical impulses by stereociliar ionic channels, which open and close due to mechanical displacements on the nanometre scale. Because of the molecular structure and asymmetric stiffness of the stereociliar bundle, the sinusoidal stimulus causes a clipped, non-sinusoidal current through the channel's transfer function of current (see Figure 6.13). In this way, the waveform is partly rectified: the electric charges flow slightly asymmetrically around the operating point, and the net movement of charges is greater into one direction. This generates a sustained depolarizing component for the time of the stimulus,

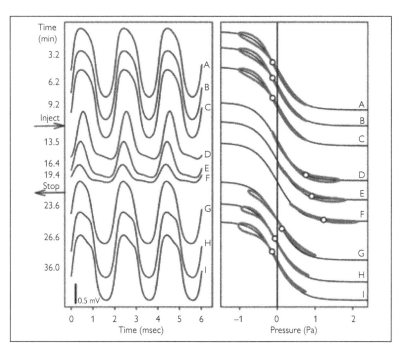

Figure 6.13 Elevated endolymphatic pressure increases distortion and asymmetry of cochlear vibration. Reversible changes during endolymphatic pressure increase elicited by gel injection ('inject'→'stop' in the middle of both panels). (left panel) Vibrations of the cochlear partition. (right panel) Shift of operating point. Reprinted from Salt *et al* (2009) © 2009, with permission from Elsevier.

following its envelope, the SP. Normally, the vibrations occur around a neutral position of the stereocilia, the so-called 'operating point', and the waveform is only slightly clipped.

Mechanically induced position changes of the organ of Corti shift the operating point (as does the gel injection in Figure 6.13), the asymmetry of the ionic fluxes; and with it, the SP increases. This is exactly what occurs in endolymphatic hydrops too. In the clinical context, the amplitude of the SP is usually compared to the action potential (AP) of the cochlear nerve. Highly asymmetrical click-evoked SP/AP values or ratios over 40% are usually considered pathologic.

Because previously only invasive Ecochg (which was done by piercing the ear drum and inserting a needle into the bony wall of the middle ear) could deliver reproducible data and also because of its supposedly low sensitivity, Ecochg has not found its way into the routine clinical test battery. Nowadays, measurements with better quality are possible even using non-invasive methods. One of the present authors has found a non-invasive variant helpful for confirming diagnosis before ablative therapy (Büki *et al* 2012). Placing a soft, wet foam electrode on the eardrum has the advantage that it can be carried out repeatedly on both ears, thereby assessing asymmetry between ears and decreasing the effect of inter-individual anatomic differences which affect both ears. With the advent of commercially available, high-tech, hand-held equipment capable of measuring Ecochg non-invasively by an ear-canal electrode, it will be possible to increase the amount of available data in the future and help to establish the place of Ecochg in the diagnostics of MD.

Other promising approaches are also emerging: it has been shown that it is possible to demonstrate abnormal pressure in the labyrinth during and after attacks by the analysis of distortion-product otoacoustic emissions phase changes during body tilt. This method is based on the principle that otoacoustic emissions are sensitive to the changes of the hair cell operating point and intracochlear pressure may simply be manipulated by body position changes (e.g. from sitting to supine position; Avan *et al* 2011).

6.3.3.3 Tests of vestibular function

In MD, at the beginning, vestibular function may be normal between attacks. Over years, when repeated attacks occur, caloric reaction frequently changes from normal to reduced, and later to absent on the affected side. The HIT usually remains normal for a long time in spite of an eventual caloric hyposensitivity. Apparently, pathological processes damage high frequency (HIT) and low frequency (caloric reaction) pathways of the vestibulo-ocular reflex (VOR) differentially.

Since the distension of the saccule usually occurs early in the course of the disease, pathologic results of otolithic tests may be anticipated. The contact of the hydropic sacculus with the stapes footplate may increase the saccular sensitivity to loud sound in some cases, thereby enhancing vestibular evoked potentials (e.g. the cervical vestibular evoked myogenic potential (cVEMP)). Later, as the disease advances, these potentials tend to disappear.

6.3.4 Differential diagnosis

Before making the diagnosis of MD, other causes, such as schwannoma of the vestibular nerve (VS), should be excluded by (gadolinium enhanced) MRI of the brain. In an advanced stage, with a history of months or years with recurrent, frequent attacks for one or two hours and unilateral hearing loss, MD usually does not pose diagnostic difficulties. At early stages, after only several attacks and a short history of weeks or months, however, differential diagnosis should include transitory ischemic attacks (TIA) of the anterior inferior cerebellar artery (AICA) territory (when age and other risk factors are present) or vestibular migraine (VM). In these latter cases, Ecochg may be of help before deciding on an ablative therapy. In recurrent BPPV, patients may sometimes relate their complaints in a way that might be interpreted as indicating MD. This may pose differential diagnostic difficulties, especially when there is an asymmetric hearing loss. Also, BPPV occurs frequently in association with MD; this has to be taken into account by the examiner.

6.3.5 Bilateral MD

It is not clear how frequently bilateral cases occur. In the literature, subsequent involvement of the contralateral ear has been reported to vary between 2% and 80% of cases. Bilateral MD poses a diagnostic and therapeutic challenge. First, one has to try to find out which side is responsible for the actual symptoms. This may be done using the anamnestic data, and Ecochg may help. Second, it is not easy to recommend an ablative therapy because vestibular function is most probably already damaged on the side of the earlier involvement, and subsequent inhibition of vestibular excitability in the second ear would certainly cause iatrogenic chronic vestibular insufficiency. However, bilateral MD may not be very frequent, and usually the attacks are not as debilitating as when there is intact contralateral vestibular function.

6.3.6 Prognosis and therapy

MD has a varying course. Periods with frequent attacks and times without any complaints may alternate. Sometimes the attacks disappear for years only to return with distressingly high frequency. The fact that spontaneous remissions are common makes the evaluation of any therapeutic effect difficult. Silverstein *et al* (1989) followed patients who were offered surgical therapy but declined. Of these patients, 57% had no complaints after two years and 71% of the patients were symptom free after an average of 8.3 years.

Many specialists prefer to try oral pharmacotherapy first, although there is no substance available which has been proven to halt the progression of hearing loss and to inhibit vertigo attacks. However, the oral therapy approach may be justified because over time many patients improve spontaneously with or without pharmacological therapy. If the disease progresses, in advanced stage (usually already with a flat hearing loss around 60–70 dB, as in Figure 6.12) frequent, severe attacks may make normal everyday life almost impossible. Two to five shorter or longer vertigo attacks in a week, with nausea and vomiting, exert a significant pressure on both the patient and the doctor. Today it is not possible to improve hearing, to stop the progression of hearing loss, or to alleviate accompanying tinnitus. However, an effective therapy for vertigo attacks is available. In MD, recurrent vertigo is caused by sudden changes of the peripheral vestibular afferent spontaneous firing rate. Since the firing rate returns to normal levels after a few hours, no central adaptation is possible. A feasible therapeutic strategy is to bring about a controlled peripheral vestibular loss in the affected ear, thereby preventing possible fluctuations of spontaneous firing rate. Earlier, when this was done by repeated injections of ototoxic aminoglycosides, deafness often occurred as a side effect. Another option previously considered—surgical ablation of the vestibular nerve—turned out to be too invasive and to cause chronic vestibular insufficiency too frequently and was therefore abandoned.

Intratympanic gentamicin therapy. In the last several years, a promising new approach has emerged in the literature: 'single injection intratympanic gentamicin therapy' (Harner *et al* 2001; Carey *et al* 2002). Evidence for the effectiveness of this method was presented in prospective, double-blind, randomized, placebo-controlled trials (Stokroos and Kingma 2004, Postema *et al* 2008). This technique uses the vestibulotoxic side effect of gentamicin. By administration of single injections of intratympanic gentamicin only when it is needed, it is possible to titrate the desired vestibular hypofunction. In this way, side effects concerning hearing (which are dose dependent) can be held on an acceptably low level (for review see Carey 2004). Gentamicin is instilled into the middle ear and kept there for 30–60 minutes (by positioning the patient in the opposite-ear-down side-lying position and instructing the patient to avoid swallowing).

Gentamicin is probably taken up by the inner ear through the round window membrane. In animal perilymph, gentamicin persists for hours after intratympanic exposure; its presence in hair cells was demonstrated for months.

Gentamycin toxicity has several different mechanisms, ranging from damage of stereocilia to mitochondrial destruction through the production of free radicals. The clinical effect, unsteadiness, develops after 2–5 days. During this short latency period, attacks may yet occur. The unsteadiness lasts for several weeks, during which time the peripheral spontaneous firing rate diminishes and a partial unilateral vestibular hypofunction develops. Then attacks do not occur any more. Some patients have strong imbalance and prefer to stay in bed for days, whereas others do not notice grave symptoms. Gentamicin causes mild inhibition of the VOR as determined by the HIT (gain reduction by 40–70%). Otolithic (saccular) function is inhibited too, as is shown by vestibular evoked potentials.

After intratympanic gentamicin administered by the single injection regimen, peripheral sensitivity remains preserved to a varying degree; there is only a **mild** peripheral vestibular deafferentation, affecting mainly type I vestibular hair cells. In chinchillas, although single intratympanic application of gentamicin caused a severe reduction in the sensitivity of SCC and otolith function, afferents nevertheless continued to fire spontaneously. Regular units had lower resting discharge rates in comparison to the contralateral side (Hirvonen et al 2005).

After a single intratympanic gentamicin injection, vertigo control is permanent in approximately 60–70% of cases, whereas in 30–40% a second injection may be needed after several months and again in one-third of the remaining cases a third injection (and so forth). In a study by de Waele et al (2002), caloric responses on the treated side returned in every third patient during the first or second year after the gentamicin injections, and the head thrust test also normalized. Half of these patients developed recurrent attacks of vertigo.

Since permanent vertigo control is not achieved in every case, Nguyen et al (2009) suggested that, to quantify percentages of patients with control of vertigo, results should be calculated, displayed, and statistically compared using the Kaplan-Meier survival calculation. They created a separate curve for each number of rounds, and failure for each was defined as the need for an additional round. This new method of visual and statistical presentation mirrors new thinking about the finely tuned 'need to do' therapy of MD, when the next injection is given only when it becomes necessary. Single injection intratympanic gentamicin is about to become the recommended state-of-the-art therapy for MD.

Ablative surgical methods (such as vestibular nerve section) are too invasive and cause side effects (such as chronic vestibular insufficiency) too frequently; other surgical manipulations (such as endolymphatic sac surgery) seem to be ineffective (e.g. Chung et al 2011).

6.4 Vestibular neuritis (VN)

VN, also called vestibular neuronitis or acute unilateral peripheral vestibulopathy, is a frequent, benign, peripheral cause of AVS, which is defined by dizziness or vertigo (with or without hearing loss) lasting more than 24 hours in the absence of focal neurologic signs. The symptoms in VN, vertigo, and vegetative complaints, are caused by a sudden, spontaneous, isolated, usually partial loss of afferent vestibular input from one labyrinth. Recently, with the advent of high resolution testing of individual SCC and otolithic organs, it has been discovered that essentially three VN subsets with different patterns exist (Aw *et al* 2001) (Table 6.3). Also, new techniques of bedside testing are available that help to differentiate between VN and potentially dangerous central causes (such as brainstem or cerebellar stroke). These developments have revived the interest of clinicians in this usually benign, peripheral vestibular disorder.

6.4.1 Pathophysiology of VN

According to widely accepted theory, VN is caused by reactivation of herpes simplex virus-1 in the vestibular ganglion cells, similar to the hypothetical pathogenic mechanism of idiopathic facial nerve palsy. According to this hypothesis, the viral inflammation leads to swelling and to a vicious circle of 'entrapment' of the nerve in the bony canal, causing collapse of the microcirculation, which in turn causes again swelling of the nerve. The acute, static symptoms are caused by the sudden decrease in the resting discharge of the afferent nerve fibres and subsequently in the vestibular nuclei on the affected side. The vestibular nerve has two divisions, and one of them or both may be affected (Table 6.3). The most common pattern is an isolated superior vestibular nerve involvement. Aw *et al* (2001) studied 33 patients with VN (29 with classic VN and 4 with simultaneous ipsilateral hearing loss). Eight patients had both the superior and inferior nerve involved; in 21 cases only the superior vestibular nerve was affected, and in two cases only the inferior nerve was involved. It has been postulated that the superior vestibular nerve is more prone to entrapment because it travels through a longer and narrower bony canal (Goebel *et al* 2001).

When in VN unilateral spontaneous firing ceases or decreases, the resulting tonic vestibular asymmetry modifies activity in all connections of the vestibular nuclei (Table 6.4).

Table 6.3 Divisions of the vestibular nerve and diagnostic methods		
Division	**Innervated structures**	**Relevant examinations showing pathological results**
Superior Nerve	Superior and horizontal SCC	Nystagmus* Caloric test Horizontal HIT (hHIT) Diagonal HIT in the RA or LA direction[†]
	Utricle (and part of the saccule)	Ocular tilt reaction (OTR)* Utricular VEMPs[†] (oVEMPs)[‡]
Inferior nerve	Inferior SCC	Sometimes slight nystagmus* Diagonal HIT in the RP or LP direction[†]
	Most of the saccule	Saccular VEMPs[†] (cVEMPs)

* Spontaneous (static) signs due to vestibular asymmetry.

[†] RA: right anterior; LA: left anterior; VEMP: vestibular evoked myogenic potential; oVEMP: ocular VEMP; RP: right posterior; LP: left posterior; cVEMPS: cervical VEMPs

Table 6.4 Symptoms and signs in VN (see also Chapters 3 and Chapter 5)	
Anatomic structure	**Result(s) of asymmetric activity**
Canal afferents to ocular motor nuclei	Spontaneous nystagmus with a fast phase to the contralateral side
Otolithic connections to cervical spinal motor neurons	Head tilt toward the side of the lesion*
Otolithic connections to ocular muscles	Vertical misalignment of the eyes and ocular counter-rolling*
Connections to lower spinal motor neurons	Veering to the side of lesion
Cerebellar connections	Downregulation of the velocity-to-position integrator: spontaneous nystagmus is more intense when looking in the direction of the fast phase (Alexander's law) Ataxic stance and gait
Connections to vegetative centres	Nausea, vomiting, sweating

* components of the OTR.

6.4.2 Symptoms

VN begins with acute spontaneous vertigo with vegetative signs and symptoms (sweating, nausea, vomiting) and postural imbalance. When the superior nerve is affected, hearing loss is lacking. It seems that the isolated neuritis of the inferior vestibular nerve may be accompanied by hearing loss (Aw et al 2001, Kim and Kim 2012).

In VN, at the beginning, the intensity of subjective vertigo increases suddenly, over hours. Although patients can stand and walk alone, they veer towards the affected side. The patients need bed rest since head movements amplify symptoms. With central compensation, symptoms gradually improve over days and weeks.

6.4.3 Diagnostic methods

6.4.3.1 Lesion of the superior and inferior vestibular nerves

When both vestibular nerve divisions are affected, static vestibular asymmetry causes horizontal-torsional spontaneous nystagmus with the fast phase beating towards the contralateral side. Each canal produces nystagmus in its own plane, and the ensuing nystagmus is the result of a three-dimensional vector summation. The purely vertical components of the nystagmus evoked by the two vertical canals neutralize each other. The torsional components from these canals are directed in the same direction, so these add to the mainly horizontal component produced by the horizontal canal.

Typical peripheral nystagmus shows a characteristic intensity change due to different gaze directions (see Section 3.3.2): it is most intensive when the patient looks towards the direction of the fast phase ('Alexander's law'). Contrary to central horizontal spontaneous nystagmus, peripheral nystagmus never changes its beating direction depending on gaze direction (as does the gaze evoked direction-changing nystagmus of central origin). Another characteristic of genuine peripheral nystagmus is that it is suppressed by fixation. Spontaneous nystagmus which is clearly seen without Frenzel's goggles should always give rise to suspicions of central spontaneous nystagmus and, conversely, patients with vertigo or dizziness should always be examined under Frenzel's goggles or similar measures (e.g. infrared video in total darkness) making fixation impossible (see Section 5.2.1.1).

When, after weeks, spontaneous nystagmus has already subsided, it can be unmasked again by head shaking and observing under Frenzel's goggles.

Other static signs of vestibular asymmetry in VN include ipsiversive OTR and veering towards the affected side when standing. From the components of the OTR (i.e. head tilt, skew deviation, and ocular torsion), head tilt and skew deviation are rarely obvious clinically in this purely peripheral entity, and if so, usually disappear quickly. Ocular torsion and deviations of the subjective visual vertical (or horizontal) may persist for a longer time.

Impaired VORs in the planes of all three ipsilateral canals in the clinical HIT and absent ipsilateral oVEMPs and cVEMPs are dynamic signs of vestibular hypofunction.

6.4.3.2 Isolated hypofunction of the superior vestibular nerve

In such cases, the ipsilateral posterior canal function and the saccular function remain intact (Figure 6.14), as they are fed into the inferior division of the vestibular nerve.

6.4.3.3 Isolated hypofunction of the inferior vestibular nerve

This entity (Halmagyi *et al* 2002) is somewhat mysterious. Its prevalence is not known, because, by causing transient dizziness and nausea without spontaneous nystagmus, it may often remain undiagnosed. Although asymmetry between the affected posterior canal and its anterior counterpart should evoke an oblique, slightly downbeating spontaneous nystagmus, there were several cases published in which little or no nystagmus was described. Also OTR and lateropulsion are absent. Auditory symptoms, however, may be present, possibly because of the close anatomical relationship between the cochlea and the inferior portion of the vestibular labyrinth.

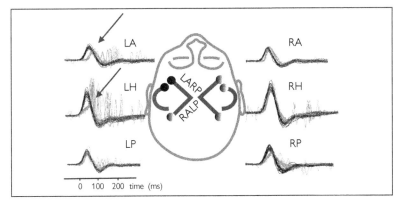

Figure **6.14** Superior nerve pattern in left-sided VN. Results of the video HIT (vHIT) in horizontal and in vertical (LARP and RALP) planes. Arrows: impaired VOR to the left in horizontal and LARP planes; the left posterior canal function is normal.

Diagnosis may be made based on a reduced VOR gain of the affected posterior SCC along with catch-up saccades and a reduced or absent saccular VEMP. Importantly, the horizontal HIT and the caloric reaction are normal. Kim and Kim (2012) found nine patients with isolated inferior neuritis out of 703 cases with the diagnosis of neuritis or labyrinthitis. This would mean that inferior neuritis is rare; however, they applied torsional downbeating nystagmus as an inclusion criterion, so they may have missed cases without spontaneous nystagmus. Of the nine patients, three also had hearing loss, and two of them showed a progression to involvement of the superior division. High-speed video goggles suitable for measuring individual vertical canal function in clinical settings will make it possible to gather more data about this elusive new entity.

6.4.4 Differential diagnosis

Chapter 2 is dedicated to the differential diagnosis of the AVS, for which VN is a frequent, clinically benign cause. Other differential diagnostic considerations should include MS, when, rarely, an isolated plaque around the nerve root entry zone develops. This causes an affection of the peripheral nerve fibres in the brain stem, before reaching central structures.

6.4.5 Prognosis and therapy

Although the function of the nerve (and excitability of the affected canals and otolithic organs with it) returns in less than half of the cases, improvement does not depend on the recovery of excitability. Symptoms due to acute static imbalance disappear with central compensation. The majority of patients do not experience disabling vertigo after one week. When function does not improve, tests of dynamic vestibular function tests (HIT, VEMPs) remain permanently pathologic.

Although vestibular suppressants may be beneficial by inhibiting strong vegetative symptoms, they hinder processes of central compensation; therefore supportive (antiemetic) therapy should be balanced between inhibiting immediate vegetative symptoms and confronting the vestibular system with the new, asymmetric situation. This confrontation can be enhanced by vestibular rehabilitation exercises, which may be started soon after the acute phase. They consist first of head movements with short, direction-changing accelerations, during which the importance of visual clues is emphasized.

It has been suggested that perhaps steroids given during the acute phase improve clinical recovery after VN (Strupp et al 2004). However, several recent reviews dispersed these hopes, as they concluded that there is currently insufficient evidence to support the administration of corticosteroids to patients with idiopathic acute vestibular dysfunction. (Goudakos et al 2010, Fishman et al 2011, Wenger et al 2102).

Following an attack of superior nerve VN, when the neuritis involves the upper part of the end-organ including the utriculus but sparing the posterior ampulla, posterior canal type BPPV may develop on the affected side. Apparently, the affected utricle releases otoconia, which then may float into the intact posterior canal.

In approximately in 20% of cases with VN, symptoms of chronic vestibular insufficiency may develop (see Chapter 7); then oscillopsia and difficulty of walking in darkness or on uneven ground are the most unpleasant symptoms.

Rarely a second or even a third relapse may occur months to years after VN; sometimes on the same side, sometimes on the other. Successive attacks are usually less pronounced than the first.

References and Further Reading

Avan P., Giraudet F., Chauveau B. *et al.* (2011) Unstable distortion-product otoacoustic emission phase in Menière's disease. *Hear Res.* **277**, 88–95.

Aw S. T., Fetter M., Cremer P. D. *et al.* (2001) Individual semicircular canal function in superior and inferior vestibular neuritis. *Neurology.* **57**, 768–74.

Aw S. T., Todd M. J., Aw G. E. *et al.* (2005) Benign positional nystagmus: a study of its three-dimensional spatio-temporal characteristics. *Neurology.* **64**, 1897–905.

Bertholon P., Bronstein A. M., Davies R. A. *et al.* (2002) Positional down beating nystagmus in 50 patients: cerebellar disorders and possible anterior semicircular canalithiasis. *J Neurol Neurosurg Psychiatry.* **72**, 366–72.

Bradshaw A.P., Curthoys I.S., Todd M.J. *et al.* (2010) A mathematical model of human semicircular canal geometry: a new basis for interpreting vestibular physiology. *J Assoc Res Otolaryngol.* **11**, 145–59.

Büki B., Ecker M., Junger H. *et al.* (2013) Vitamin D deficiency and benign paroxysmal positioning vertigo. *Medical Hypotheses.* **80**, 201–4.

Büki B., Jünger H., Avan P. (2012) Cochlear function in Ménière's disease. *Int J Audiol.* **51**, 373–8.

Büttner U., Helmchen C., Brandt T. (1999) Diagnostic criteria for centralversus peripheral positioning nystagmus and vertigo: a review. *Acta Otolaryngol.* **119**, 1–5.

Carey J. (2004) Intratympanic gentamicin for the treatment of Meniere's disease and other forms of peripheral vertigo. *Otolaryngol Clin North Am.* **37**, 1075–90.

Carey J. P., Hirvonen T., Peng G. C. *et al.* (2002) Changes in the angular vestibulo-ocular reflex after a single dose of intratympanic gentamicin for Ménière's disease. *Ann N Y Acad Sci.* **956**, 581–4.

Chung J. W., Fayad J., Linthicum F. *et al.* (2011) Histopathology after endolymphatic sac surgery for Ménière's syndrome. *Otol Neurotol.* **32**, 660–4.

De Waele C., Meguenni R., Freyss G. *et al.* (2002) Intratympanic gentamicin injections for Meniere disease: vestibular hair cell impairment and regeneration. *Neurology.* **59**, 1442–4.

Epley J. M. (1992) The canalith repositioning procedure: for treatment of benign paroxysmal positional vertigo. *Otolaryngol Head Neck Surg.* **107**, 399–404.

Fishman J. M., Burgess C., Waddell A. (2011) Corticosteroids for the treatment of idiopathic acute vestibular dysfunction (vestibular neuritis). *Cochrane Database Syst Rev.* CD008607.

Goebel J. A., O'Mara W., Gianoli G. (2001) Anatomic considerations in vestibular neuritis. *Otol Neurotol.* **22**, 512–8.

Goldberg J. M. (2000) Afferent diversity and the organization of central vestibular pathways. *Exp. Brain Res.* **130**, 277–97.

Goudakos J. K., Markou K. D., Franco-Vidal V. *et al.* (2010) Corticosteroids in the treatment of vestibular neuritis: a systematic review and meta-analysis. *Otol Neurotol.* **31**, 183–9.

Hallpike C.S. and Cairns H. (1938) Observations on the Pathology of Ménière's Syndrome: (Section of Otology). *Proc R Soc Med.* **31**, 1317–36.

Halmagyi G. M., Aw S. T., Karlberg M. *et al.* (2002) Inferior vestibular neuritis. *Ann N Y Acad Sci.* **956**, 306–13.

Halmagyi G. M., Weber K. P., Curthoys I. S. (2010) Vestibular function after acute vestibular neuritis. *Restor Neurol Neurosci.* **28**, 37–46.

Harner S. G., Driscoll C. L., Facer G. W. *et al.* (2001) Long-term follow-up of transtympanic gentamicin for Ménière's syndrome. *Otol Neurotol.* **22**, 210–4

Hirvonen T. P., Minor L. B., Hullar T. E. *et al.* (2005) Effects of intratympanic gentamicin on vestibular afferents and hair cells in the chinchilla. *J Neurophysiol.* **93**, 643–55.

Jeong S. H., Kim J. S., Shin J. W. *et al.* (2012) Decreased serum vitamin D in idiopathic benign paroxysmal positional vertigo. *J Neurol.* **260**, 832–8.

Kim J. S. and Kim H. J. (2012) Inferior vestibular neuritis. *J Neurol.* **259**, 1553–60.

Lundberg Y. W., Zhao X., Yamoah E. N. (2006) Assembly of the otoconia complex to the macular sensory epithelium of the vestibule. *Brain Res.* **1091**, 47–57.

Merchant S. N., Adams J. C., Nadol J. B. Jr. (2005) Pathophysiology of Meniere's syndrome: are symptoms caused by endolymphatic hydrops? *Otol Neurotol.* **26**, 74–81.

Merchant S. N., Velázquez-Villaseñor L., Tsuji K. *et al.* (2000) Temporal bone studies of the human peripheral vestibular system. Normative vestibular hair cell data. *Ann Otol Rhinol Laryngol Suppl.* **181**, 3–13.

Minor L. B., Schessel D. A., Carey J. P. (2004) Méniére's disease. *Curr Opin Neurol.* **17**, 9–16.

Monsell E. M., Balkany T. A., Gates G. A. *et al* (1995) Goldenberg RA, Meyerhoff WL, House JW: Committee on Hearing and Equilibrium guidelines for the diagnosis and evaluation of therapy in Meniere's disease. *Otolaryngol Head Neck Surg.* **113**, 181–5.

Nguyen K. D., Minor L. B., Della Santina C. C. *et al.* (2009) Time course of repeated intratympanic gentamicin for Ménière's disease. *Laryngoscope.* **119**, 792–8.

Oghalai J. S., Manolidis S., Barth J. L. *et al.* (2000) Unrecognized benign paroxysmal positional vertigo in elderly patients. *Otolaryngol Head Neck Surg.* **122**, 630–4.

Perez P., Franco V., Cuesta P. *et al.* (2012) Recurrence of benign paroxysmal positional vertigo. *Otol Neurotol.* **33**, 437–443.

Postema R. J., Kingma C. M., Wit H. P. *et al.* (2008) Intratympanic gentamicin therapy for control of vertigo in unilateral Meniere's disease: a prospective, double-blind, randomized, placebo-controlled trial. *Acta Otolaryngol.* **128**, 876–80.

Rabbitt R. D., Yamauchi A. M., Boyle R. *et al.* (2001) How endolymph pressure modulates semicircular canal primary afferent discharge. *Ann N Y Acad Sci.* **942**, 313–21.

Ross M. D., Peacor D., Johnsson L. G. *et al.* (1976) Observations on normal and degenerating human otoconia. *Ann Otol Rhinol Laryngol.* **85**, 310–26.

Salt A.N., Brown D.J., Hartsock J. J. *et al.* (2009) Displacements of the organ of Corti by gel injections into the cochlear apex. *Hear Res.* **250**, 63–75.

Salt A. N., Inamura N., Thalmann R. *et al.* (1989) Calcium gradients in inner ear endolymph. *Am J Otolaryngol.* **10**, 371–5.

Salt A. N. and Plontke S. K. (2010) Endolymphatic hydrops: pathophysiology and experimental models. *Otolaryngol Clin North Am.* **43**, 971–83.

Savastano M., Guerrieri V., Marioni G. (2006) Evolution of audiometric pattern in Meniere's disease: long-term survey of 380 cases evaluated according to the 1995 guidelines of the American Academy of Otolaryngology-Head and Neck Surgery. *J Otolaryngol.* **35**, 26–9.

Schuknecht H. F. (1963) Meniere's disease: a correlation of symptomatology and pathology. *Laryngoscope.* **73**, 651–665.

Silverstein H., Smouha E., Jones R. (1989) Natural history vs. surgery for Menière's disease. *Otolaryngol Head Neck Surg.* **100**, 6–16.

Stokroos R. and Kingma H. (2004) Selective vestibular ablation by intratympanic gentamicin in patients with unilateral active Ménière's disease: a prospective, double-blind, placebo-controlled, randomized clinical trial. *Acta Otolaryngol.* **124**, 172–5.

Strupp M., Zingler V. C., Arbusow V. *et al.* (2004) Methylprednisolone, valacyclovir, or the combination for vestibular neuritis. *N Engl J Med.* **351**, 354–61.

Teranishi M., Yoshida T., Katayama N. *et al.* (2009) 3D computerized model of endolymphatic hydrops from specimens of temporal bone. Acta *Otolaryngol Suppl.* **560**,43–7.

Thalmann R., Ignatova E., Kachar B. *et al.* (2001) Development and maintenance of otoconia: biochemical considerations. *Ann N Y Acad Sci.* **942**, 162–78.

Uzun-Coruhlu H., Curthoys I. S., Jones A. S. (2007) Attachment of the utricular and saccular maculae to the temporal bone. *Hear Res.* **233**, 77–85.

Vibert D., Kompis M., Häusler R. (2003) Benign paroxysmal positional vertigo in older women may be related to osteoporosis and osteopenia. *Ann Otol Rhinol Laryngol.* **112**, 885–9.

Wegner I., van Benthem P. P., Aarts M. C. *et al.* (2012) Insufficient Evidence for the Effect of Corticosteroid Treatment on Recovery of Vestibular Neuritis. *Otolaryngol Head Neck Surg.* **147**, 826–31.

Yamakawa, K. (1938). Pathologic changes in a Meniere's patient. *J Otolaryngol Jpn.* **44**, 2310–12.

Chapter 7

Chronic vestibular insufficiency

Key points

- Chronic vestibular insufficiency (CVI) is caused by dysfunction of peripheral vestibular structures (hair cells, vestibular nerve), leading to an afferent deficit.
- It is usually the result of bilateral vestibular deafferentation (BVD); however, sometimes severe unilateral vestibular hypofunction may elicit similar symptoms.
- Complaints include gait unsteadiness that becomes worse in darkness and on uneven ground, oscillopsia with head movements, and impaired spatial orientation.
- The most frequent causes of BVD are vestibulotoxic antibiotics (such as gentamicin) and bilateral Menière's disease (MD). However, up to 50% of cases remain idiopathic.
- In BVD, the head impulse test (HIT) is highly positive with overt compensatory saccades, results of dynamic visual acuity testing are pathologic, and patients cannot stand on a foam mat with closed eyes.

7.1 Introduction

CVI is usually caused by BVD; sometimes, however, unilateral vestibular loss, e.g. vestibular neuritis (VN) or unilateral neurectomy, causes CVI (see Table 7.1). After BVD, vestibulo-ocular reflexes (VORs) are permanently deficient, but postural stability and posturally-related cardiovascular responses recover over time. 'Vestibular compensation' is a general term for the neural mechanisms instrumental in regaining balance and postural coordination after vestibular loss. It allows the restoration of near normal spontaneous neural activity in the ipsilesional vestibular nucleus. In this way, the resting discharge activities of the left and right vestibular nuclei are rebalanced, which parallels the clinical recovery. With acute bilateral lesions, however, activity in the vestibular nuclei decreases on both sides; hence, spontaneous activity has to be raised bilaterally. Apparently, in this process non-labyrinthine sensory inputs 'from above and below' have an important role (for review see McCall and Yates 2011). The term 'from below' indicates that nerve impulses obtained from somatosensory inputs and visceral graviceptors deliver inputs mainly to the caudal vestibular nuclei.

Table 7.1 Causes of CVI	
• *Idiopathic*	• 50% of cases
• *Unilateral vestibular hypofunction*	• VS[†] or its operation
	• After VN
• *Bilateral vestibular hypofunction*	• Ototoxic antibiotics (gentamycin alone or in combination with other ototoxic drugs)[*]
	• Ototoxic chemotherapeutics (e.g. cisplatin)
	• Bilateral MD
	• Neuropathies (B_{12} deficiency, HSMN IV[†], neurosarcoidosis)
	• Neurodegenerative disorders (SCA, EAII, MSA, SAOA, CANVAS)[†]
	• Autoimmune systemic/inner ear disease
	• CJD[†]
	• Cogan's syndrome
	• NF2[†] with bilateral acoustic neurinoma
	• Haemosiderosis
	• Meningoencephalitis
	• Bilateral traumatic vestibulopathy

[*] Renal insufficiency was described as an additional toxicity risk factor for antibiotics due to systemic accumulation.
[†] Abbreviations: CANVAS: cerebellar ataxia, neuropathy, vestibular areflexia syndrome; CJD: Creutzfeldt-Jakob disease; EAII: episodic ataxia type 2; HSMN IV: hereditary sensory and autonomic neuropathy; MSA: multiple system atrophy; NF2: Neurofibromatosis Type 2; SAOA: sporadic adult-onset ataxia of unknown origin; SCA: spinocerebellar ataxia; VS: vestibular schwannoma.

The term 'from above' indicates that descending inputs from the cerebral cortex play a larger role in regulating the excitability of neurons in the rostral vestibular nuclei. For example, Fetsch *et al* (2010) showed that neurons in the primate dorsal medial superior temporal area compute vestibular responses and are thus involved in the integration of visual and vestibular signals to facilitate perception of self-motion, similar to the brainstem and thalamus. Animal experiments suggest that for vestibular compensation after BVD—and subsequent recovery of behavioural and motor responses—the increased integration of such non-labyrinthine inputs in the central vestibular system is essential.

Why some patients fully recover after an acute vestibular lesion and others do not is still debated. Missing somatosensory inputs in neuropathies, cerebellar pathologies, and impaired vision make compensation almost impossible. Other factors that usually interfere with recovery include advanced age, medical interventions, immobility, and psychosocial problems. CVI may either gradually worsen over time or present with an acute onset, for example after application of ototoxic substances or due to meningitis. In about one-third of cases, episodic vertigo precedes chronic symptoms. Patients with slowly progressive CVI may notice few complaints, probably because there is time for the central compensation to evolve. BVD is rare amongst vestibular disorders, accounting for only 4% (Zingler *et al* 2007). However, the impact of BVD on the quality of life is considerable, with two-thirds of patients reporting slight or moderate impairment. Establishing the diagnosis of BVD is often delayed by years.

7.2 Complaints and clinical findings

Oscillopsia (i.e. apparent motion of the visual scene) on fast head turns, ataxic gait while walking in the dark or on uneven ground, and impaired spatial orientation are key clinical findings in patients with CVI.

Whereas gait unsteadiness can be found in almost all CVI patients (99%), oscillopsia during active (fast head turns, walking) or passive head movements is less frequently reported (44%) (Zingler *et al* 2007). Symptoms in CVI will be most prominent when compensatory strategies, i.e. relying more on vision and proprioception, fail, such as during walking on uneven ground, in darkness, or when wearing shoes with thick soles. In healthy subjects, the VOR compensates for head perturbations during walking, allowing a stable gaze, e.g. while reading a street sign or recognizing faces. Bilateral impairment of the VOR will force these patients to stop in order to read the sign or recognize a face; otherwise, retinal slip will lead to oscillopsia. When at rest, typically no complaints are reported.

Clinical examination should focus on the identification of unilateral or bilateral vestibular hypofunction, other neurological signs, and associated findings. Use of the standard Romberg test (feet together, eyes closed) may not be sensitive enough to detect CVI. Reducing proprioception at the same time, either by standing on a soft surface (e.g. a foam mat) or by placing the feet heel-to-toe may unmask more discrete increases in postural sway. The examiner must be aware that patients with CVI may fall when applying this test, as both vestibulo-spinal reflexes and compensatory visual and proprioceptive input are lacking. However, increased sway may also be related to peripheral polyneuropathy (PNP) affecting the lower extremities, underlining the necessity to search for signs of PNP in these patients. In the clinical examination, the HIT is the single most important test when vestibular insufficiency is suspected. It will reliably identify patients with compensatory late (or 'overt') catch-up saccades as sign of vestibular hypofunction. However, a presumably normal clinical (bedside) HIT does not exclude unilateral or bilateral vestibular hypofunction—as the hypofunction might be more discrete or as patients might generate early ('covert') compensatory saccades that require a quantitative assessment of the HIT (e.g. by use of video-oculography). Another bedside test of the VOR is the dynamic visual acuity test (DVA). It compares distant visual acuity with the head still (i.e. static) and when oscillating the patient's head (i.e. dynamic) manually (with frequencies around 2 Hz). A DVA of three or more lines above static visual acuity indicates a vestibular defect (see Figure 7.1).

If history taking and clinical examination suggest a diagnosis of CVI, it should be confirmed by laboratory audio-vestibular testing. Ideally, this includes assessing the SCCs both at high (vHIT, DVA) and low (rotation, caloric irrigation) frequencies, the otolith organs (cervical vestibular evoked myogenic potential (cVEMP), ocular vestibular evoked myogenic potential (oVEMP)), hearing (pure tone audiometry), and postural stability (dynamic posturography). While most patients with BVD will have deficits at both high and low head rotation frequencies, isolated high-frequency or low-frequency impairments are sometimes found. Neurological signs pointing towards cerebellar

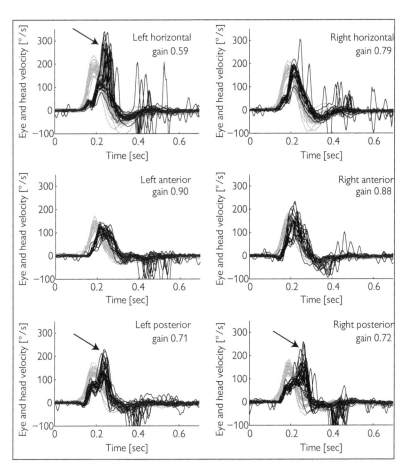

Figure 7.1 Video HIT (vHIT) of all six semicircular canals (SCCs) in a patient with a partially recovered bilateral vestibular deficit after antibiotic treatment with gentamicin 3.5 years ago. The grey traces refer to the applied head impulses; the resulting compensatory eye velocity traces are indicated by the black traces. At the time of testing, the patient still noticed blurred vision mainly on head turns to the left and upward (but not downward). These clinical complaints nicely match the findings in the vHIT, with patchy loss of vestibular function of the left horizontal and both posterior canals, as reflected by early (covert) catch-up saccades (indicated by arrows) and a reduced gain for the left horizontal canal (0.59, cut-off > 0.75). This case underlines the clinical utility/value of measuring both horizontal and vertical canals.

disease (such as limb ataxia, downbeat-nystagmus, dysarthria), asymmetrical hearing loss with a suspected tumour in the cerebello-pontine angle, Cogan syndrome, or autoimmune disease should prompt brain magnetic resonance imaging (MRI). Likewise, head computed tomography (CT) should be ordered when there is suspicion for transverse temporal bone fracture. A laboratory work-up may be needed if autoimmune disease is considered.

7.3 Aetiology of vestibular hypofunction

If the history, clinical examination, and vestibular testing confirm vestibular hypofunction, the diagnostic approach aims to identify the underlying cause to eventually provide the patient with a suitable treatment (if available).

7.3.1 Bilateral vestibular hypofunction as a cause of CVI

A definite or probable cause of BVD was found in 49% of cases, leaving 51% undiagnosed (Zingler et al 2007). The most frequent causes of BVD (Black 2010) include antibiotics-related ototoxicity. In this group, gentamicin deserves special consideration. It is a common misconception that the ototoxicity of gentamicin may be monitored by pure tone audiometry. Being dominantly vestibulotoxic and acting with a latency of days and even weeks, systemic gentamicin may cause subtle bilateral vestibular ablation, which is already irreversible at the time of its identification. It appears that there is no safe dose level for the vestibular system (Halmagyi et al 1994). In many patients, even therapeutically correct dosage may cause CVI if there is coexisting renal impairment. After a treatment in intensive care, the effects of vestibular loss may not become apparent until mobilization. Indication of systemic gentamicin therapy should take into account these complications and it should be reserved for life-saving therapies when other antibiotics (such as 4th-generation cephalosporines) are not available. Other causes include anti-cancer chemotherapeutic agents (1–4%), bilateral MD (7–15%), trauma (bilateral temporal bone fracture, <10%), meningoencephalitis (5–11%), neuropathies (1–9%), tumours (e.g. neurofibromatosis type II, 1–2%), neurodegenerative disorders (spinocerebellar ataxia, multiple system atrophy (MSA), cerebellar degeneration, 4–13%), and autoimmune disorders (sarcoidosis, Sjögren's syndrome, Behcet's disease, 1–9%). Recurrent VN seems to be rare (2% recurrence rate over ten years; Zingler et al 2007). Associated neurological disorders were noted in 39% of BVD patients (Rinne et al 1998). Whereas PNP may be found in 22% of cases, another study found evidence for BVD in 38% of patients with confirmed PNP. A cerebellar syndrome can be observed in up to 25% of BVD patients, with additional PNP in one-third of these patients (Zingler et al 2007). Bilateral hypoacusis was found in 25% of BVD patients and was associated mostly with primary otological disorders.

7.3.2 Unilateral vestibular hypofunction as a cause of CVI

Typical symptoms of CVI occur in about 20% of cases with unilateral hypofunction. After vestibular neurectomy, even if only unilateral, CVI often develops. The most frequent causes of CVI after unilateral vestibular hypofunction include acute VN or labyrinthitis, MD, post-traumatic vestibulopathy, and labyrinthine ischaemia. Onset is often abrupt, and vestibular hypofunction usually marked, leading to intense symptoms (vertigo, nausea, oscillopsia, gait imbalance) and clear clinical signs (e.g. spontaneous nystagmus, pathologic HIT).

7.4 Treatment and prognosis

Whenever possible, a directed treatment against the underlying condition should be applied. This, however, is possible only in a minority of patients for two main reasons: a diagnosis can be made only in half of the CVI patients, and some of them may have suffered irreversible structural damage. If feasible, vestibulotoxic antibiotics should be replaced by non-vestibulotoxic substances. Similarly, anti-cancer chemotherapeutics leading to hair cell damage should be avoided in the future. A diagnostic work-up for the underlying cause of concomitant polyneuropathy is mandatory and may lead to a treatment (e.g. vitamin B_{12} supplementation, alcohol abstinence) that may be beneficial for the vestibular organs also. If no directed treatment is possible, optimizing the other sensory systems involved in balance and spatial orientation is important to improve central compensation. This includes intensive, regular, and early vestibular exercises and balance training, ophthalmologic visits, and tight control of blood glucose levels in diabetics. Gait is improved in about 50% of patients after regular and structured vestibular rehabilitation over the period of 3–12 months. Patients are also advised to wear shoes with slim soles, use a walking aid, and avoid the intake of sedatives as they may increase complaints. Immunosuppressive treatment may be necessary in patients with autoimmune disorders.

With 50% idiopathic CVI cases and limited treatment options, prognosis in CVI is often unfavourable: in a follow-up study with clinical re-evaluation after a mean of 51 months, more than 80% of BVD patients did not improve (Zingler *et al* 2008), including all cases related to ototoxic antibiotics. Prognosis is favourable in most cases with acute-onset unilateral vestibular deficits; however, functional recovery may take months and may be incomplete. In cases of CVI due to unilateral vestibular hypofunction, sometimes spontaneous recovery of peripheral function occurs.

There is no correlation between the extent of the persisting peripheral vestibular deficit as measured for example with the HIT and the extent of disability due to CVI experienced by patients when peripheral vestibular function does not fully recover after acute VN (Palla *et al* 2008).

7.5 **Precautions to avoid/limit CVI**

Our understanding of CVI is far from complete. Nonetheless, an underlying cause is identified in every second patient, providing important insights into the mechanisms causing or facilitating the occurrence of CVI. Recommendations include restricted use of aminoglycosides and, if possible, treatment of the underlying cause of CVI (e.g. vitamin B_{12} deficiency). If the administration of vestibulotoxic antibiotics is required, reassurance should be made about a normal renal function, and a combination with other potentially ototoxic substances (e.g. furosemide) must be avoided. Also, baseline vestibular testing should be performed prior to the administration of potentially vestibulotoxic drugs, and bedside vestibular testing is mandatory at follow-up visits (including bedside HIT and DVA). In patients with polyneuropathy, treatable disorders should be identified and corrected.

References and Further Reading

Black F. O. (2010) Acquired bilateral peripheral vestibulopathy. In: Eggers S. D Z., Zee D. S. (eds), Vertigo and Imbalance: Clinical Neurophysiology of the Vestibular System. Handbook of Clinical Neurophysiology, Vol. 9. Elsevier B.V. pp. 333–52.

Fetsch C. R., Rajguru S. M., Karunaratne A. *et al.* (2010) Spatiotemporal Properties of Vestibular Responses in Area MSTd. *J Neurophysiol* **104**, 1506–22.

Halmagyi G. M., Fattore C. M., Curthoys I. S. *et al.* (1994) Gentamicin vestibulotoxicity. *Otolaryngol Head Neck Surg.* **111**, 571–4.

Halmagyi G. M., Weber K. P., Curthoys I. S. (2010) Vestibular function after acute vestibular neuritis. *Restor Neurol Neurosci.* **28**, 37–46.

McCall A. A. and Yates B. J. (2011) Compensation following bilateral vestibular damage. *Front Neurol.* **2**, 88.

Palla A., Straumann D., Bronstein A. M. (2008) Vestibular neuritis: Vertigo and the high-acceleration vestibulo-ocular reflex. *J Neurol.* **255**, 1479–82.

Rinne T., Bronstein A. M., Rudge P. *et al.* (1998) Bilateral loss of vestibular function: clinical findings in 53 patients. *J Neurol.* **245**, 314–21.

Wiest G., Demer J. L., Tian J. *et al.* (2001) Vestibular function in severe bilateral vestibulopathy. *J Neurol Neurosurg Psychiatry.* **71**, 53–7.

Zingler V. C., Cnyrim C., Jahn K. *et al.* (2007) Causative factors and epidemiology of bilateral vestibulopathy in 255 patients. *Ann Neurol.* **61**, 524–32.

Zingler V. C., Weintz E., Jahn K. *et al.* (2008) Follow-up of vestibular function in bilateral vestibulopathy. *J Neurol Neurosurg Psychiatry.* **79**, 284–8.

Chapter 8

Diseases of the temporal bone and schwannoma of the vestibular nerve

Key points

- Diseases of the temporal bone may elicit fluctuating changes in the spontaneous firing rate of the vestibular nerve or cause permanent vestibular deafferentation.
- Clinical signs of temporal bone fractures include bleeding from the outer ear canal or blood behind the eardrum and, in cases of labyrinthine or neural damage, signs of unilateral cochleovestibular deafferentation and/or facial nerve palsy.
- A pathological third labyrinthine window causes pseudoconductive hearing loss and fluctuating dizziness or vertigo due to pressure or sound-related movements of the perilymph.
- Since vestibular schwannoma (VS) most frequently presents with unilateral sensorineural hearing loss as a first symptom, every case of sudden or slowly evolving asymmetric sensorineural hearing loss should be evaluated by (at least non-contrast) magnetic resonance imaging (MRI) of the brain.

8.1 Diseases of the temporal bone

8.1.1 Introduction

Diseases of the temporal bone may cause permanent, one-time transient or fluctuating changes of vestibular nerve resting discharge. Permanent, usually unilateral deafferentation occurs with fractures or overt bacterial inflammation of the inner ear; transient dysfunction is seen in patients with labyrinthine concussion or successfully treated bacterial labyrinthitis. Chronic fluctuating vestibular activity is usually elicited by the pathological behaviour of one of the existing windows, such as in cases with rupture of the round window membrane (see Chapter 12) or with pathological movements of the stapes. Sometimes, vestibular dysfunction is caused by a pathological third window of the inner ear, which opens towards the intracranial spaces, thereby allowing the transmission of pressure changes or sound-evoked endolymph movements in the direction of the highly sensitive vestibular hair cells.

8.1.2 Temporal bone diseases causing permanent peripheral deafferentation

8.1.2.1 Temporal bone fractures

Approximately 80% of all temporal bone fractures run longitudinally through the temporal bone, usually anterior to the otic capsule, that is anterior to the region of the dense bone immediately surrounding the inner ear, thus sparing the inner ear (for review see Johnson et al 2008). Approximately every second longitudinal fracture involves the middle ear and causes dislocation of the ossicles, resulting in conductive hearing loss. Transverse fractures (approximately 10%) travel perpendicular to the long axis of the petrous pyramid generally involving the otic capsule. In approximately 10% of cases, the fracture shows both longitudinal **and** transverse aspects. The two different fracture types involve the bony canal of the facial nerve with similar frequency. Recently, new, more clinically oriented classifications have been suggested, such as 'otic capsule violating' vs 'otic capsule sparing' or 'petrous' vs 'nonpetrous'. These classifications seem to correlate better with complications such as leak of cerebrospinal fluid (CSF), sensorineural hearing loss, vertigo, and facial nerve lesion.

If the fracture line runs along the outer ear canal or through the middle ear, clinical signs of temporal bone fracture are bleeding from the outer ear canal or blood behind the eardrum, as well as perforation of the eardrum. In cases of labyrinthine or neural damage, signs of unilateral cochleovestibular deafferentation, such as vertigo, hearing loss, facial nerve palsy, and spontaneous nystagmus, appear. Imaging should be done with high-resolution computed tomography (CT) of the temporal bone. The acute signs of vestibular deafferentation improve with central compensation.

8.1.2.2 Infections

Infections of the external or middle ear, which may involve the inner ear, usually do not pose diagnostic problems because of the characteristic symptoms such as pain (e.g. in malignant external otitis caused by Pseudomonas aeruginosa in elderly patients with diabetes mellitus), discharge (chronic otitis media), or eruptions in the external auditory canal (herpes zoster oticus). Chronic cholesteatoma, causing perhaps only a small perforation on the eardrum but major hidden destruction even without discharge and hearing loss, may only be seen by otomicroscopy.

8.1.2.3 Otosclerosis

In this disorder of bone metabolism unique to the otic capsule, focal bone resorption and rebuilding of spongiotic bone cause conductive or combined hearing loss by fixating the stapes in the oval window. Sensorineural hearing loss at some frequencies is common; vertigo and dizziness (recurrent, positional, or spontaneous) occur in 30–40 % of patients with otosclerosis, often with permanently decreased caloric excitability. It has been suggested that sensorineural hearing loss and vestibular signs and symptoms could be due to changes in the biochemical composition of the perilymph. The mechanism of this, possibly toxic, dysfunction is unknown (for a review see Baloh and Kerber 2011; Coreoglu et al 2010).

8.1.3 Temporal bone diseases causing fluctuating peripheral vestibular activity

The labyrinth and its fluid-filled space, the perilymphatic space, is connected to the surrounding fluid- and air-filled spaces by two windows and two canals. Two broad and mobile windows open towards the middle ear (the oval window with the stapes in it and the round window, which equalizes inner ear fluid pressure changes during stapes displacements); two long and narrow canals connect the labyrinth with the intracranial (subarachnoidal) space: the cochlear aqueduct and the vestibular aqueduct (with the endolymphatic duct within; for a review see Merchant and Rosowski 2008). Other microscopic connections contain nerves and blood vessels.

When a third window opens on the inner ear, hearing loss and balance problems may emerge. This may occur due to developmental failure or when one of the existing two windows becomes highly mobile or leaking.

8.1.3.1 Symptoms and signs

Positive fistula-test: vertigo and nystagmus caused by pressure variation in the external meatus in cases with eardrum perforation and chronic otitis media.

Hennebert's sign: vertigo and nystagmus caused by pressure variations in the ear canal with **an intact eardrum**.

Tullio phenomenon: vertigo and nystagmus induced by loud sounds. It is usually caused by a pathological window on one of the semicircular canals (SCCs) that allows shunting of compressive pressure waves from the stapes towards the intracranial space. Intracranial pressure changes (e.g. pressing against the closed glottis) may also elicit vertigo in patients with canal dehiscence; however, the description 'Tullio phenomenon' is reserved for loud **sounds** eliciting vertigo.

Conductive hearing loss: intact hearing threshold with bone-conducted stimulation but elevated threshold when using air-conducted stimuli.

8.1.3.2 Endolymphatic hydrops/Hypermobile stapes syndrome

In patients with increased endolymphatic pressure/volume, the membrane of the saccule may touch the inner surface of the stapes (see upper panel of Figure 6.10). In that case, or when the stapes footplate moves with an abnormally large amplitude (usually after footplate-fractures or ear operations), pressure changes in the external ear canal elicit deformations of the membranous labyrinth, causing dizziness and eye movements. Hennebert's sign was primarily described in cases of congenital syphilis (caused possibly by syphilitic hydrops). Today it is most frequently seen in Menière's disease (MD).

8.1.3.3 Erosion of the lateral canal

A cholesteatoma may destroy the horizontal SCC wall and create a pathological opening of the canal towards the middle ear (Figure 8.1). This allows for pressure changes in the external meatus to be transmitted directly onto the membranous labyrinth (fistula sign). Patients may experience vertigo during the Valsalva manoeuvre against closed nostrils.

8.1.3.4 Syndromes of the 'third mobile window'

Large additional openings of the inner ear towards the intracranial spaces, such as canal dehiscences and large vestibular aqueducts, may shunt the energy of air-conducted

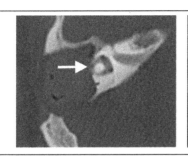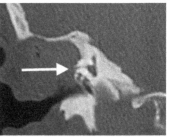

Figure 8.1 Cholesteatoma destroying the horizontal SCC. Left panel: axial CT scan of the right temporal bone; the white arrow laid over the cholesteatoma matrix shows the opening on the SCC. Right panel: coronal CT scan. Image by courtesy of Dept. of Radiology, County Hospital Krems an der Donau, Austria.

sounds away from the cochlea (Merchant and Rosowski 2008) (see Figure 8.2). Instead of moving the basilar membrane, which is very stiff around the oval window, sound pressure escapes through the broad connection in the direction of the intracranial space, thereby elevating air-conduction thresholds. However, when stimuli are presented by bone vibrators, the additional broad connection increases the deformability of the otic capsule by permitting movements of the incompressible perilymph: bone-conduction thresholds will be even lower than in normals. There is an increased difference between a better bone conduction and worse air conduction: an air-bone gap with an intact eardrum ensues. Since an air-bone gap with a normal eardrum is much more common in cases of otosclerosis, care must be taken to differentiate between the two to avoid unnecessary stapes surgery. In otology, an air-bone gap is always a sign for a conductive blockage in the middle ear and an indication for middle ear surgery for improving hearing; in cases with a third mobile window, however, a 'pseudoconductive' hearing loss develops. The cause of this is in the inner ear and, understandably, an operation does not improve the situation.

SCCD. Patients with SCCD complain of vertigo and oscillopsia evoked by loud noises and/or by manoeuvres changing intracranial pressure (such as coughing, sneezing, or straining against closed glottis). Auditory complaints include autophony (hearing one's own voice loudly), hypersensitivity to bone-conducted sounds, such as noises originating in the patient's own body (e.g. noises elicited by eye movements) and conductive hearing loss on audiometry. Sometimes vestibular symptoms dominate, in other cases both auditory and vestibular manifestations can be demonstrated; occasionally patients have only auditory complaints. When first describing this syndrome, Minor *et al* (1998) demonstrated that the eye movements were aligned with the plane of the affected canal when stimulated by sound or manoeuvres that caused labyrinthine pressure changes. In a histopathologic study carried out on 1000 temporal bones of unselected human subjects, Carey *et al* (2000) found frank dehiscence in 0.5% and thin bone (less than 0.1 mm) in 1.4%. Bilateral dehiscence was frequent. There were no vestibular symptoms noted in the corresponding clinical records. Infants had thin bone over the superior canal in the middle fossa at birth, with gradual thickening until three years of age. Hagiwara (*et al* 2012) found *radiologic* SCCDs in every fourth (!) child

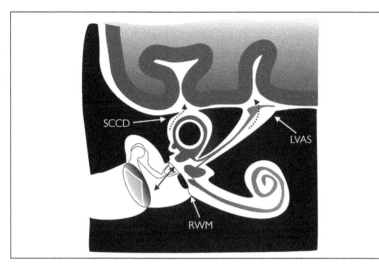

Figure 8.2 The mechanisms of leaking pressure waves as suggested by Merchant and Rosowski (2008). SCCD: semicircular canal dehiscence; LVAS: large vestibular aqueduct syndrome; RWM: round window membrane; double arrow: stapes movements; dotted arrows: routes of escaping pressure waves.

less than two years of age and in 3% of adults. Nadgir et al (2011) found a statistically significant increase in the prevalence of radiographic dehiscence as age increased (in the elderly over 60 years of age). Apparently, radiological dehiscence is common, histological dehiscence is rare, and cases with manifest symptoms are even less frequent. In childhood, the labyrinth is often more exposed; later in life, development thickens the bone above the canals. In old age, thinning of the bone may occur again (see Figure 8.3).

Diagnosis of SSCD. Instrumental examinations may help to clarify the diagnosis and to differentiate SCCD from otosclerosis. In spite of the air-bone gap at low and middle frequencies (< 2000 Hz) the acoustic reflex remains intact in SCCD, but not in otosclerosis. Cervical vestibular evoked potential (cVEMP) testing shows lower-than-normal thresholds (Zhou et al 2012). This latter result seems to be especially useful, since cVEMPs otherwise reliably disappear with real conductive hearing loss. High-resolution CT scans reconstructed in the plane of the suspected canal and orthogonal to this plane may deliver additional information, which has to be evaluated in context with the clinical findings. In the literature, in cases with debilitating symptoms, operative resurfacing of the canal has brought improvement.

Large vestibular aqueduct syndrome (LVAS). The vestibular aqueduct, containing the endolymphatic duct, runs from the vestibule to the posterior cranial fossa. Its (usually bilateral) congenital enlargement causes auditory and vestibular symptoms (for a review see Berrettini et al 2005; Gopen et al 2011). On audiometry, it presents usually with combined hearing loss of varying severity, with a low frequency pseudoconductive component similar to that in SCCD. In spite of the air-bone gap, air-conducted cVEMP and middle ear reflex testing may show normal results. This should raise the

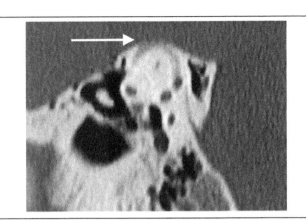

Figure 8.3 CT scan of a dehiscence on the superior SCC. Arrow: dehiscence on the cranial part of the SCC; the scan was done in the plane of the right superior canal. Image by courtesy of Dept. of Radiology, County Hospital Krems an der Donau, Austria.

suspicion of a third window, since these methods are very sensitive to threshold elevation due to ossicular fixation. In children, LVAS is found frequently in cases with otherwise unexplained sensorineural hearing loss (in approximately 30%). During life, sensorineural hypoacusis sometimes fluctuates and progresses; in other cases it remains constant. Minor head trauma, large sudden shifts of barometric pressure, or Valsalva manoeuvres seem to accelerate progression. Considering that the tips of the cochlear hair cell stereocilia register displacements of several nanometres (!) under physiological circumstances around hearing threshold, intracranial pressure waves may possibly harm hearing when they are transmitted relatively unhindered on the highly sensitive structures of basilar membrane. Because of the possible damaging effects of trauma, some clinicians even recommend restricting activities, such as contact sports, to decrease the possibility of hearing loss associated with head trauma. Vestibular symptoms (episodic vertigo, unsteadiness, and peripheral hypofunction) have been reported by different authors to occur with a frequency between 0–100% (see the review of Gopen *et al* 2011) depending on different selection criteria and variable length of follow-up.

LVAS may be isolated or a feature of a complete Mondini deformation (a highly variable congenital dysplasia of the cochlea or the inner ear, looking as if development would have been arrested at the 7th week of gestation). When Mondini dysplasia is associated with postpuberty goiter, this is the Pendred syndrome, an autosomal recessive disorder caused by a mutation of the PDS gene. It is characterized by the missing anion exchanger protein pendrin, which is involved in the cellular transport of chloride, iodine, and bicarbonate anions. Clinical and radiological signs of LVAS should prompt evaluation of thyroid function to shed light on undiagnosed, mild thyroid symptoms (Berrettini *et al* 2005).

Apart from clinical signs such as normal ear drum, (pseudo-)conductive hearing loss, intact air-conducted cVEMP (eventually with lower thresholds than normal) and normal

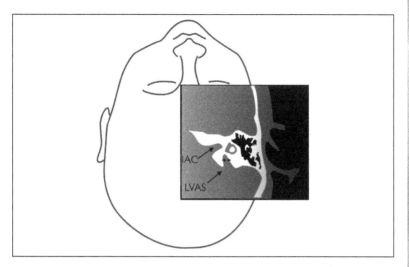

Figure 8.4 Schematic drawing of the radiological presentation of LVAS on an axial CT scan. LVAS: abnormally large vestibular aqueduct; IAC: internal auditory canal; horizontal double arrow: the aperture is usually measured around the middle of the aqueduct.

middle ear reflex thresholds, diagnosis of LVAS requires demonstration of enlarged aqueduct on axial CT scans of the temporal bone (e.g. a diameter larger than 1.5 mm midway between the outer aperture and common crus) or on high-resolution MRI.

Because of the progressive hearing loss, in many cases cochlear implantation may be necessary (see Figure 8.4).

8.2 Vestibular schwannoma (VS)

Although other usually benign lesions (such as meningeoma) may also grow in the cerebellopontine angle, VS is the most frequent. It causes a slow unilateral (in neurofibromatosis often bilateral) cochleovestibular deafferentation. The most frequent primary complaints are unilateral hearing loss and tinnitus. There are usually no acute vestibular symptoms, because the central vestibular compensation keeps pace with the slowly developing asymmetry of afferent discharge. Therefore, chronic imbalance and dizziness are the most frequent vestibular complaints. However, sometimes patients complain of true vertigo attacks, which last for hours or are fluctuating for days. Hearing loss may progress slowly, but sometimes develops suddenly. It may fluctuate or even transiently improve; therefore, in every case of sudden hearing loss or newly diagnosed unilateral sensorineural hearing loss/tinnitus, radiologic workup is indicated. For radiologic screening, non-contrast MRI seems to be sufficient. Since MRI is widely available and cost-efficient, the measurement of auditory brainstem responses is no longer considered as the primary test to screen for VS (Fortnum et al 2009). Gadolinium-contrasted T1-weighted MRI sequences are recommended in cases of suspected pathology.

Currently, there are no universally accepted, evidence-based clinical practice treatment guidelines for VS. Treatment decision algorithms to decide between the three possible strategies ('wait and scan', operation, or radiosurgery) include the following factors: initial tumour diameter, increase of tumour size over time, initial hearing level, age, and health of the patient, eventual brainstem compression, patient's choice, and experience of the clinician. During surgery of small tumours, complete tumour removal and preservation of hearing may be a goal in addition to conservation of intact facial nerve function. If operation is not possible or recommended, fractionated stereotactic radiotherapy may bring about long-term or permanent tumour regression.

Based on the studies of hereditary types of schwannoma, in the last few years, promising new molecular therapy modalities have emerged (for a review see Terry and Plotkin 2012).

Hereditary neurofibromatosis includes two types, both inherited in an autosomal dominant fashion. The more common neurofibromatosis type 1 (NF1 or Recklinghausen's disease), with mainly cutaneous tumours, is caused by a mutation on the 17th chromosome for a protein also known as neurofibromin. The less frequent neurofibromatosis type 2 (NF2) has been linked to mutations of the *NF2* gene on the 22nd chromosome, resulting in deficiency of merlin (moesin-ezrin-radixin-like protein), a tumour suppressor, also called schwannomin. This mutation causes schwannomas, meningiomas, retinal hamartomas, and ependymomas. In cells gathered from operated **sporadic** VS, merlin was also deficient. Apparently, loss of merlin decreases contact-dependent inhibition in Schwann cells by inhibiting the epidermal growth factor receptor (EGFR). Merlin deficiency may result in an abnormal activation of receptor tyrosine kinases (RTKs). An oral human epidermal growth factor receptor (HER)-1/EGFR tyrosine kinase inhibitor has already been approved for the treatment of non–small cell lung cancer and pancreatic cancer. After showing promising results in animal experiments in preliminary studies, the agent also slowed tumour growth rate in patients with NF2 and progressive VS, exhibiting a cytostatic effect on merlin-deficient cells (Terry and Plotkin 2012).

Vascular endothelial growth factor (VEGF) is a mediator of angiogenesis and vascular permeability. VEGF and the VEGF receptor 1 (VEGFR1) have been detected in sporadic and NF2-associated schwannomas, with increased levels correlating with increased rates of tumour growth. In animal experiments, anti-VEGF monoclonal antibodies, approved for the treatment of various cancers, often in combination with traditional chemotherapeutic drugs, can increase apoptosis, reduce tumour growth rate, and increase survival in rodents with intracranial schwannomas.

References and Further Reading

Baloh R. W. and Kerber K. A. (2011) Clinical neurophysiology of the vestibular system. Oxford University Press, New York.

Berrettini S., Forli F., Bogazzi F. *et al.* (2005) Large vestibular aqueduct syndrome: audiological, radiological, clinical, and genetic features. *Am J Otolaryngol.* **26**, 363–71.

Carey J. P., Minor L. B., Nager G. T. (2000) Dehiscence or thinning of bone overlying the superior semicircular canal in a temporal bone survey. *Arch Otolaryngol Head Neck Surg.* **126**, 137–47.

Cureoglu S., Baylan M. Y., Paparella M. M. (2010) Cochlear otosclerosis. *Curr Opin Otolaryngol Head Neck Surg.* **18**, 357–62.

Fortnum H., O'Neill C., Taylor R. *et al.* (2009) The role of magnetic resonance imaging in the identification of suspected acoustic neuroma: a systematic review of clinical and cost effectiveness and natural history. *Health Technol Assess.* **13**, 1–154.

Gopen Q., Zhou G., Whittemore K. *et al.* (2011) Enlarged vestibular aqueduct: review of controversial aspects. *Laryngoscope.* **121**, 1971–8.

Hagiwara M., Shaikh J. A., Fang Y. *et al.* (2012) Prevalence of radiographic semicircular canal dehiscence in very young children: an evaluation using high-resolution computed tomography of the temporal bones. *Pediatr Radiol.* **42**, 1456–64.

Johnson F., Semaan M. T., Megerian C. A. (2008) Temporal bone fracture: evaluation and management in the modern era. *Otolaryngol Clin North Am.* **41**, 597–618.

Merchant S. N. and Rosowski J. J. (2008) Conductive hearing loss caused by third-window lesions of the inner ear. *Otol Neurotol.* **29**, 282–9.

Minor L. B., Solomon D., Zinreich J. S. *et al.* (1998) Sound- and/or pressure-induced vertigo due to bone dehiscence of the superior semicircular canal. *Arch Otolaryngol Head Neck Surg.* **124**, 249–58.

Nadgir R. N., Ozonoff A., Devaiah A. K. *et al.* (2011) Superior semicircular canal dehiscence: congenital or acquired condition? AJNR *Am J Neuroradiol.* **32**, 947–9.

Terry A. R. and Plotkin S. R. (2012) Vestibular Schwannoma: Evidence-based Treatment. Chemotherapy: present and future. *Otolaryngol Clin North Am.* **45**, 471–86.

Wong H., Lahdenranta J., Kamoun W. *et al.* (2010) Anti-vascular endothelial growth factor therapies as a novel therapeutic approach to treating neurofibromatosis-related tumors. *Cancer Res.* **70**, 3483–93.

Zhou G., Poe D., Gopen Q. (2012) Clinical use of vestibular evoked myogenic potentials in the evaluation of patients with air-bone gaps. *Otol Neurotol.* **33**, 1368–74.

Chapter 9

Central causes of vertigo, dizziness, and imbalance

Key points

- Recurrent dizzy spells unexplained by other central or peripheral vestibular abnormalities and with a history of migraine headaches are the basis for a diagnosis of migraine-associated vertigo or dizziness.
- Vertebrobasilar stroke is the most frequent central cause of acute vestibular syndrome (AVS), defined as acute-onset vertigo or dizziness lasting >24 hours, accompanied by nausea/vomiting, head-motion intolerance, nystagmus, and gait imbalance.
- Brief attacks of vertigo or dizziness accompanied by other brainstem or cerebellar signs suggest a vertebrobasilar transient ischaemic attack (TIA).
- Vertigo, dizziness, and various abnormalities in the execution of voluntary movements (ataxia) are frequent complaints in multiple sclerosis (MS).
- While 10% of central-type AVS is related to MS, the most frequent cause of episodic vertigo in MS remains a coincidental benign paroxysmal positional vertigo (BPPV).
- Cerebellar ataxia presents with ataxia of gait/stance and of the extremities, dysarthria, and ocular motor abnormalities.
- Ataxia of gait/stance and of the extremities in combination with spasticity and increased tendon reflexes suggest sensory ataxia related to myelopathy, whereas peripheral neural dysfunction and loss of tendon reflexes point to neuropathy.
- Important causes for both myelopathy and neuropathy include vitamin B_{12} deficiency, paraneoplastic syndromes, and neurosyphilis.
- Wernicke's encephalopathy (WE), alcohol or drug intoxication, and cerebellar stroke present as acute-onset ataxia.
- Paraneoplastic cerebellar degeneration, MS, and Creutzfeldt-Jakob disease (CJD) are important differential diagnoses for subacute onset of ataxia.
- Cerebellar degeneration due to chronic alcohol consumption, multiple system atrophy (MSA), and sporadic adult-onset ataxia are the most frequent disorders associated with slowly progressive sporadic ataxia.
- Whereas most autosomal-recessive ataxias become symptomatic under 20 years of age, autosomal-dominant ataxias, including spinocerebellar ataxias (SCAs) and episodic ataxias (EAs), may emerge later in life.

(Continued)

Spinocerebellar ataxia type 6 (SCA6) may be responsible for up to 20% of progressive adult-onset cerebellar ataxias.

- If the diagnostic work-up (magnetic resonance imaging (MRI), genetic testing) in adult-onset ataxia remains negative, sporadic adult-onset ataxia is diagnosed, but regular follow-up is nevertheless mandatory. Accompanying severe orthostatic hypotension will support a diagnosis of cerebellar type MSA (MSA-C).
- Treatment with acetazolamide and 4-aminopyridine (4-AP) may significantly reduce oscillopsia, vertigo, and ataxia in sporadic adult-onset ataxia, SCA6, and episodic ataxia type 2 (EA2).
- Dizziness and vertigo are frequent complaints in epileptic seizures, either related to epileptic aura or anti-epileptic drug-induced side effects.
- Pure vertical or torsional positional nystagmus should cast doubt on a diagnosis of peripheral BPPV, especially if repetitive liberation manoeuvres remain ineffective.
- There is no certain sign or examination by which it is possible to differentiate between central or peripheral positional nystagmus.

9.1 **Introduction**

In cases with dizziness or vertigo, normal findings in peripheral vestibular testing or signs of focal neurological deficits turn the examiner's focus on a possible central origin of complaints. However, the distinction as to whether complaints are 'peripheral' or 'central' may be challenging, and the consequences are major. In this situation, a structured approach to the wide range of disorders potentially related to 'central' dizziness, vertigo, or imbalance is needed.

Therefore a detailed but focused history taking and bedside examination are indispensable, frequently followed by neuroimaging. Whereas dizziness or vertigo is common in many central disorders, it is often non-specific and may be related to the treatment subsequently initiated. Those patients mainly complaining of gait imbalance rather than vertigo or dizziness may have an underlying sporadic, degenerative, or inherited cause, which needs further evaluation.

9.2 **Vestibular migraine (VM)**

VM (migraine-associated vertigo, migraine-associated dizziness, migraine-related vestibulopathy) is defined as vertigo or dizziness caused by migraine (Eggers 2007).

9.2.1 **Epidemiology**

Migraine is recognized as a frequent cause of central dizziness or vertigo in young and middle-aged patients. There are no internationally approved diagnostic criteria available; therefore it is difficult to gather exact epidemiological data. It seems that the prevalence of migraine is higher in those individuals with dizziness than in the general population and that patients with migraine often complain of dizziness or vertigo. The lifetime prevalence of VM has been estimated at 1% of the population (Neuhauser and Lempert 2009).

VM is more common in females and often runs in the family, probably with an autosomal-dominant pattern of inheritance. VM does not fulfil the diagnostic criteria for basilar migraine since other posterior circulation aura symptoms, apart from vertigo/dizziness, are missing. As for migraine headaches, VM does not have any specific biologic markers; therefore its diagnosis has to rely on the patient's clinical complaints. In most patients, the typical migraine headaches start earlier in life than the vestibular symptoms. There may even be a symptom-free interval lasting years between the disappearance or reduction of migraine headaches and the onset of vestibular symptoms (typically in the 30s to 40s). Not infrequently, migraine headaches are replaced by episodic dizziness or vertigo in women around the menopause. The pathophysiology of VM may be related to cortical spreading depression within the multisensory vestibular temporo-parietal regions; however, several acute findings, including peripheral vestibular hypofunction or nystagmus, cannot be explained by cortical dysfunction.

9.2.2 Diagnostic approach for VM

The diagnostic criteria of VM (Neuhauser and Lempert 2009) do not require the simultaneous occurrence of migraine headaches and dizzy spells. 'Probable' and 'definitive' types of VM have been suggested (see Table 9.1), the latter accounting only for one-third of VM patients. VM may present with many different faces, which is probably best demonstrated in the range of duration of the dizzy spells, falling within the typical

Table 9.1 Diagnostic criteria for 'definitive' and 'probable' VM (Neuhauser and Lempert 2009)

Definitive VM

A) Episodic vestibular symptoms of at least moderate severity*
B) Current or previous history of migraine according to the 2004 criteria of The International Headache Society (IHS)
C) One of the following migrainous symptoms during two or more attacks of vertigo[§]:

   migrainous headache, photophobia, phonophobia, visual aura, or other aura

D) Other causes ruled out by appropriate investigations

Probable VM

A) Episodic vestibular symptoms of at least moderate severity*
B) One of the following:
   (1) current or previous history of migraine according to the 2004 criteria of the IHS;
   (2) migrainous symptoms during vestibular symptoms[§];
   (3) migraine precipitants of vertigo in more than 50% of attacks: food triggers, sleep irregularities, or hormonal change; or
   (4) response to migraine medications in more than 50% of attacks
C) Other causes ruled out by appropriate investigations

* Vestibular symptoms are 'moderate' if they interfere with but do not prohibit daily activities and 'severe' if patients cannot continue daily activities.

[§] In the diagnostic criteria, vestibular symptoms were restricted to rotations or other illusory self- or object-motion, whereas dizziness was not considered a criterion. Whether this distinction is justified remains an open issue. The symptoms may be spontaneous or positional.

range of aura symptoms (5–60 minutes) only in a minority of patients. Spells range from seconds (10%) to minutes (30%) and hours (30%) to days (30%), and recovery from an attack may take weeks. Some patients even report persistent dizziness. Lack of triggers is characteristic, as is the history of migraine headaches, a tendency for kinetosis, and the duration of spells (usually minutes to hours). VM episodes may be accompanied by migraine-type headaches, vegetative symptoms, photophobia, and phonophobia, as well as osmophobia. It has been suggested, however, that they can occur also without other migraine-related symptoms. Headaches are often less intense than the 'usual' migraine headaches and accompany at least some episodes of vertigo/dizziness in 30–70% of patients, with the temporal relation to headaches often being variable.

Patients with VM typically complain of spontaneous vertigo or dizziness; however, positional dependence is found in 40–70% of cases examined. Whereas in BPPV positional vertigo lasting 5–20 seconds is characteristic, in VM, vertigo is persistent. In the differential diagnosis, the identification of other migraine-associated features, such as visual or other aura symptoms, photophobia or phonophobia, and migraine-specific precipitants (i.e. menstruation, sleep irregularities, stress, specific food, and sensory stimuli), is important as they may present the only apparent link between the dizziness/vertigo and migraine.

The clinical examination in migraine patients often shows minor abnormalities, such as, for example, a vibration-induced nystagmus (without evidence for a vestibular deficit in the head impulse test (HIT)) or a pronounced end-point nystagmus (without other cerebellar signs). Hearing loss and tinnitus are infrequent (but their presence may make the distinction from Menière's disease (MD) or an anterior inferior cerebellar artery (AICA) stroke more difficult). Peripheral vestibular hypofunction on caloric irrigation is noted in 10–20% of VM patients, but is also found in patients with 'classic' migraine headaches without vertigo or dizziness. Brain imaging in the patient with suspected VM is indicated when complaints are newly developed or when the patient reports an increase or change of symptoms. Since VM is often a diagnosis by exclusion, repeated positional testing (to exclude BPPV), audiometry and electrocochleography (Ecochg; to exclude MD), and radiologic examination (cerebral MRI) should be carried out in order to eliminate other differential diagnostic entities. Reduction of complaints under prophylactic therapy (see Section 9.2.4) may confirm the diagnosis.

9.2.3 Differential diagnosis

The most important differential diagnoses are MD (search for hearing problems), vertebrobasilar TIA or stroke (search for focal neurological signs), central positional vertigo (CPV) or BPPV, episodic motion sickness and—much less frequently—EA2 (look for cerebellar signs). Whereas stroke is typically suspected in elderly patients, vertebral artery dissection leading to ischaemia may be mistaken for VM or vertebrobasilar migraine in younger individuals. Migraine seems to be associated with other disorders leading to dizziness and vertigo such as MD and BPPV, EA2, and motion sickness. Prevalence of migraine is twice as high in patients with MD compared to healthy subjects; migraine is two times more likely in patients with idiopathic BPPV than in matched controls.

Table 9.2 Treatment of acute VM attacks*
NSAID as Naproxen 500 mg or Ibuprofen 400–800 mg
Aspirin 500–1000 mg
Paracetamol 1000 mg
Compound analgesics
Triptans, oral (e.g. sumatriptan 25–50 mg, naratriptan 2.5 mg, zolmitriptan 2.5–5 mg), nasal (zolmitriptan 2.5–5 mg, sumatriptan 20 mg) or injectable (sumatriptan 6 mg) formulations
Ergotamine derivatives

* add antiemetics (e.g. domperidone, metoclopramide) if required

9.2.4 Treatment options for VM

The decision for acute and prophylactic treatment depends both on the severity of single attacks and its frequency. Specific treatment recommendations (see Tables 9.2 and 9.3) for VM are scarce and are based on expert opinion and small case series only. Use of the same treatment strategies that are effective in migraine headaches for treating VM seems justified. Note that dizziness or vertigo in migraine patients may also be related to drug treatment. Beta-blockers may lead to orthostatic hypotension, and antidepressants or anti-epileptic drugs may lead to imbalance, sleepiness, and dizziness.

A re-evaluation of the response to prophylactic treatment should be made after three months. A reduction in the attack frequency of 50% or more can be considered a realistic goal.

9.3 Cerebrovascular disorders leading to central vertigo/dizziness

Cerebrovascular disorders may result in dizziness or vertigo by various mechanisms. Again, history taking is essential to distinguish transient symptoms (as in TIA) from prolonged complaints (as in stroke) and to identify accompanying neurological symptoms. In all cases, urgent referral to the emergency department (ED), ideally followed by further treatment in a specialized stroke unit, is essential. Symptom onset is typically abrupt in dizziness or vertigo related to cerebrovascular causes, and some complaints (e.g. gait imbalance or vomiting) may be excessively intensive compared to the others (e.g. severe vomiting accompanied by mild gait imbalance).

9.3.1 Vertebrobasilar stroke

About 18% of all ischaemic strokes affect the posterior circulation, and about 50–70% of those are associated with dizziness or vertigo as the presenting or prominent symptom (Tarnutzer et al 2011). Vertebrobasilar ischaemic stroke counts for about 80% of central causes of AVS, defined as acute-onset vertigo or dizziness lasting 24 hours or more, accompanied by nystagmus, nausea or vomitus, unsteady gait, and intolerance

Table 9.3 Treatment options for VM (based on data from Goadsby and Sprenger 2010; Silberstein *et al* 2012)	
Prophylactic treatment*	Side effects
Beta-blocker	
• Propranolol 40–240 mg/d (Level A)	Fatigue, hypotension, impotence, depression, bronchospasm
• Metoprolol 50–200 mg/d (Level A)	Fatigue, hypotension, impotence, depression, bronchospasm
Anticonvulsants	
• Topiramate 50–200 mg/d (Level A)	Cognitive impairment, weight loss
• Valproat 800–1200 mg/d (Level A)	Drowsiness, weight gain, tremor, haematological and liver abnormalities
Antidepressants	
• Amitriptyline 25–75 mg/d (Level B)	Sedation, anticholinergic side effects, conduction block
• Venlafaxine 75–150 mg/d (Level B)	Cardiac arrhythmia, drowsiness, urinary retention
Calcium channel blocker	
• Flunarizine 5–10 mg/d	Weight gain, sedation, depression
Diuretics	
• Acetazolamide 250–750 mg/d (Level U)	Paraesthesia, nausea, sedation, hypokalaemia, hyperglycaemia
Non-pharmaceutical treatments	
• Magnesium 30 mmol/d (titrate)	Diarrhoea
• Vitamin B_2 (Riboflavin) 400 mg/d	
• Coenzyme Q_{10} 150–300 mg/d	Gastrointestinal complaints
Lifestyle modifications	
• Avoidance of triggers, regular sleep	
• Regular physical exercise	
• Vestibular physiotherapy	

* Classification of recommendations (after Silberstein *et al* 2012; see Appendix for definition of Class I–IV studies):

A: Established as effective, ineffective, or harmful (or established as useful/predictive or not useful/predictive) for the given condition in the specified population. (Level A rating requires at least two consistent Class I studies)

B: Probably effective, ineffective, or harmful (or probably useful/predictive or not useful/predictive) for the given condition in the specified population. (Level B rating requires at least one Class I study or two consistent Class II studies).

U: Data inadequate or conflicting; given current knowledge, treatment (test, predictor) is unproven.

to head motion. Whereas age is a risk factor for cerebrovascular disease along with other vascular risk factors (hypertension, dyslipidaemia, smoking and a positive family history for stroke, myocardial infarction, or peripheral arterial disorders), vertebral artery dissection (VAD) may be the underlying cause in younger patients and must be specifically searched for in strokes before age 50 (Gottesman *et al* 2012). Typically, dizziness or vertigo lasts more than 24–48 hours when caused by stroke. Up to 30% of stroke patients report brief prodromal episodes of dizziness or vertigo in the weeks to months before vertebrobasilar stroke. After a first TIA, the risk for a subsequent stroke is highest within the first 90 days. Whereas prolonged dizziness or vertigo presenting along with focal neurological symptoms and signs as numbness, diplopia, Horner syndrome, or hemiataxia is a strong predictor for posterior fossa pathology, isolated AVS (i.e. without obvious focal neurological signs) may be falsely associated with a more benign peripheral disorder, such as acute vestibular neuritis (VN). Probably up to 50% of patients with central AVS do not show any obvious focal neurological signs (Tarnutzer et al 2011). The distinction between peripheral and central causes of isolated acute dizziness/vertigo is therefore important to identify those patients that need close monitoring and urgent treatment.

9.3.1.1 Vascular anatomy of the posterior circulation

The main vessel in the posterior circulation (see Figure 3.8), the basilar artery (BA), emerges from the fusion of the two ascending vertebral arteries. Its most important branches are the posterior inferior cerebellar artery (PICA, emerging from the vertebral arteries), the AICA (branching off the lower part of the BA), and the superior cerebellar artery (SCA) originating from the upper part of the BA. The three paired vessels that provide the blood supply for the cerebellum (PICA, AICA, and SCA) also supply the lateral brainstem by their proximal branches. Therefore signs of brainstem stroke are commonly found in patients with cerebellar stroke (Lee 2009). Depending on the affected vessel, different clinical syndromes with acute dizziness/vertigo (73%), nausea or vomiting (54%), gait disturbances (48%), and headache (37%) emerge (Edlow et al 2008). Note that ischaemia may affect two or more vessels (e.g. combined AICA and PICA stroke), resulting in more extensive lesions.

Key findings in cerebellar stroke include ataxia (limbs or trunk, 50–60%), dysarthria (46%), nystagmus (horizontal gaze-evoked and direction-changing or vertical, 44%) and confusion (26%). Whereas ischaemia in the territory of the PICA is more common than SCA stroke, ischaemia in the AICA territory is least frequently found (for detailed clinical vascular syndromes see Edlow et al 2008). Importantly, the vascular anatomy shows developmental variations in up to 50% of patients in the posterior circulation, resulting in distinct clinical presentations in individuals affected. For example, the internal auditory artery originates from the PICA (instead the AICA) in rare cases.

Stroke in the posterior circulation is most frequently related to atherosclerosis and subsequent stenosis or occlusion of the feeding vessels or to embolic (cardiac or arterial origin) disorders. Emboli in the posterior circulation preferentially occlude distal arterial branches supplying the cerebellum. Searching for an embolic source is therefore important in patients with isolated cerebellar stroke, which accounts for about 3% of all strokes.

9.3.1.2 PICA stroke

Blood supply for the lateral medulla (including the vestibular nuclei) and the postero-inferior cerebellum (including the inferior vermis) is provided by the PICA. Ischaemia in the distal PICA (e.g. at the level of the medial branch) may result in isolated AVS without auditory symptoms, whereas more proximal occlusions will present with partial or complete Wallenberg syndrome (i.e. ipsilateral hemiataxia, trigeminal sensory loss, Horner syndrome, contralateral crossed sensory loss, and hiccoughs). The result of a three-step bedside test, consisting of the **H**ead **I**mpulse test, searching for direction-changing **N**ystagmus and **T**est of **S**kew deviation (HINTS, see Chapter 2) is highly sensitive and specific in PICA strokes (Figure 9.1) limited to the cerebellum (Tarnutzer *et al* 2011), as the brainstem anatomical structures responsible for the vestibulo-ocular reflex (VOR) remain intact. However, incomplete Wallenberg syndrome including the vestibular nuclei can present as vestibular pseudoneuritis with an ipsilaterally positive HIT (Figure 9.2).

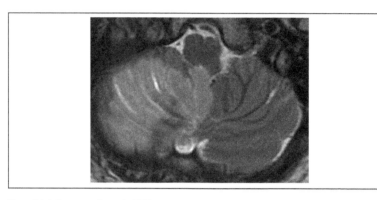

Figure 9.1 Ischaemic stroke in the PICA territory in a patient presenting with prolonged vertigo, repetitive vomiting, and gait ataxia. On clinical examination, slight gaze-evoked nystagmus on right-gaze was noted, whereas the horizontal HIT (hHIT) was normal, and no skew deviation was found, suggesting a central origin of AVS. As no obvious focal neurological signs were present, this case is consistent with a diagnosis of isolated central AVS. MRI image courtesy of the Department of Neuroradiology, University Hospital Zurich, Switzerland.

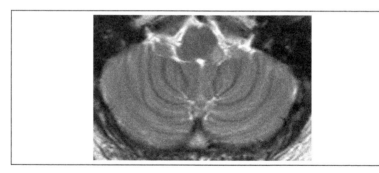

Figure 9.2 Partial Wallenberg Syndrome on the left side, including the left vestibular nuclei, presumably due to left VAD. This 61-year-old patient presented with left neck pain, followed by acute prolonged vertigo and impaired gait. He also reported slight left-sided facial numbness and clumsiness with the left hand. On examination, spontaneous right-beating nystagmus, a catch-up saccade on the HIT to the left, slight dysmetria of the left hand, and discrete left sided trigeminal hypaesthesia were found. Initially, this patient was diagnosed with acute VN; however, based on the duplex sonography (demonstrating no flow in segments V0-3 of the left vertebral artery) and the MRI, the diagnosis was revised. MRI image courtesy of the Medizinisch Radiologisches Institut, Zurich, Switzerland.

9.3.1.3 AICA stroke

Occlusion of the AICA typically results in combined labyrinthine (supplied by the internal auditory artery), cerebellar (flocculus, anterior inferior cerebellum), and brainstem (posterolateral pons including the vestibular nuclei, middle cerebellar peduncle) ischaemia, presenting with a pattern of combined peripheral (labyrinthine) and central (brainstem and cerebellar) signs and symptoms. Due to either ischaemia of the labyrinth or of the vestibular nuclei in AICA stroke, the hHIT is typically pathological, suggesting a peripheral-type lesion (e.g. acute VN). In these cases, the clinician must search for other clues pointing to a central origin, including ocular motor findings according to the HINTS test, sudden unilateral hearing loss (present in about 60% of AICA strokes), and additional brainstem signs (e.g. hemiataxia, abducens palsy, facial palsy, and Horner syndrome).

9.3.1.4 SCA stroke

Ischaemia within the territory of the SCA affects both brainstem (posterolateral midbrain) and cerebellar structures (superior cerebellum including the dentate nucleus). Cerebellar lesions in SCA stroke result in acute imbalance and dysarthria, nausea, and vomiting. As in AICA and PICA stroke, vertigo or dizziness may accompany SCA stroke, although its frequency seems to be lower.

9.3.1.5 Diagnostic approach in vertebrobasilar stroke

Distinguishing dangerous and potentially life-threatening central causes from more benign peripheral causes can be achieved more reliably with the three-step bedside ocular motor examination HINTS than with brain MRI, including diffusion-weighted imaging (DWI), within the first 24–48 hours. Any of the dangerous HINTS pointing to INFARCT (Impulse Normal, Fast-phase Alternating, Refixation on Cover Test) predicts a central cause with high sensitivity. In case of an initially negative MRI (including DWI) and clinical signs and symptoms suggestive of a central cause of AVS, repeating the MRI three to ten days after first symptoms is recommended, as MRI within the first 24 to 48 hours may be negative in approximately 20% of stroke patients. Whereas non-contrast cranial computer-tomography (CCT) identifies acute intracranial haemorrhage reliably, its sensitivity for the diagnosis of acute ischaemic stroke is 40% or less (Hwang et al 2012). Focusing on the posterior fossa in AVS and due to the fact that only about 4% of central AVS cases are caused by haemorrhage, the diagnostic yield of CCT in the assessment of dizziness/vertigo in the ED is low.

Whereas combined cerebellar and brainstem strokes are usually readily identified by the clinician, it is the isolated cerebellar syndromes presenting only with non-specific symptoms, such as nausea or vomiting and subtle ocular motor signs, that may be difficult to recognize as a stroke. The most important differential diagnoses in AVS related to stroke are other central (e.g. demyelination within the brainstem including the vestibular nuclei, VM) and peripheral (e.g. acute VN) causes.

Both a mass effect of the stroke itself or an underlying cause of VAD may lead to head or neck pain in addition to dizziness or vertigo in vertebrobasilar stroke. In AVS, headache is present in probably about 30–40% of patients and is more frequent with central-type AVS (Tarnutzer et al 2011). The combination of pain and dizziness may complicate the differential diagnosis, especially in the young: this is because craniocervical pain and prolonged dizziness or vertigo are frequent complaints both in VM and (extracranial) VAD leading to vertebrobasilar stroke, which represents a larger proportion of stroke causes in patients before the age of 50 than after. With the most frequent complaints in VAD (vertigo or dizziness (58%), headache (51%), and neck pain (46%)) being unspecific (Gottesman et al 2012), the clinician may find the distinction between migraine and stroke difficult. In such situations, the intensity of the headache may help differentiate migraine from VAD: whereas headaches in VM are often mild, craniocervical pain in VAD tends to be sudden, sustained (lasting more than three days), and severe. Preceding minor trauma increases the likelihood of VAD by a factor of about four; however, absence of (even minor) head or neck trauma does not exclude the possibility of VAD, as trauma is present in less than half of VAD patients.

In patients with confirmed vertebrobasilar stroke, further diagnostics (a search for large vessel stenosis, occlusion, or some other source of embolic disease), monitoring, and treatment should be provided in a specialized stroke unit. Delayed diagnosis of vertebrobasilar, but especially cerebellar stroke may result in fatal—although treatable—complications, such as obstructive hydrocephalus, mass effect from oedema formation, brainstem compression, and recurrent stroke. In cases of cerebellar stroke, 10–20% of patients deteriorate (indicated by i.e. a subsequently developing gaze palsy or progressive worsening of the level of consciousness) in the days following the event, with swelling peaking on the third day after infarction. Thus, patients whose AVS is mistakenly thought to be due to a peripheral vestibular cause (if dizziness or vertigo is predominant) or due to a non-vestibular cause, such as a migraine headache, acute gastroenteritis (if vomiting is the presenting symptom), or intoxication, may appear to be clinically stable at the time of discharge from the ED but at risk of severe complications days later.

9.3.1.6 Therapy

Proposed recanalization treatments in acute vertebrobasilar stroke include systemic and local thrombolysis and stenting. These procedures, however, are still experimental, and guidelines are lacking. In cases of progressive cerebellar oedema, external ventricular drainage and/or suboccipital craniotomy (including removal of the infarcted tissue) may be considered. Whereas cerebellar stroke with a subsequent comatose state results in death in 85% of cases if untreated, craniotomy may lead to a good outcome (modified Rankin scale score of two or less) in about 50% of cases (Edlow et al 2008). Steroids have no effect on the oedema related to ischaemia.

9.3.2 Vertebrobasilar TIA

A brief episode of dizziness, vertigo, or hearing impairment (usually lasting for minutes) may precede either vertebrobasilar stroke (representing vertebrobasilar TIAs) or acute VN within a few days, and this phenomenon has been observed to occur in the same percentage of cases (25%) for both conditions. However, repetitive episodes noted over a period of weeks to months favour an ischaemic origin over an inflammatory one. If triggered by head rotations, the differential diagnosis of rotational vertebral artery syndrome (RVAS) should be considered, whereas a postural dependence may point to a haemodynamically relevant stenosis in the vertebrobasilar circulation. Transient diplopia, incoordination, extremity weakness, and sudden falls are the most frequent accompanying signs of vertebrobasilar TIA. The differential diagnosis of transient dizziness or vertigo is broad and includes other dangerous causes, such as cardiac arrhythmia or hypoglycaemia. If triggered by positional changes, causes more frequent than vertebrobasilar TIA should be searched for, primarily BPPV and orthostatic hypotension; but in addition, dangerous mimics, such as internal bleeding leading to hypotension and anaemia and CPV, need to be considered. If triggered by head turns or when wearing neck collars or ties, carotid sinus hypersensitivity may also be a differential diagnosis. Because 5% of TIA patients suffer a stroke within 48 hours, prompt diagnosis is critical. Even in the absence of large vessel occlusion in the posterior circulation, the risk of stroke within the first 90 days after TIA is approximately 20%. Overall, vertebrobasilar TIA presents a rare but dangerous cause of transient central dizziness/vertigo. Accompanying symptoms (hearing loss, migraine headache) and signs (focal neurological signs, drop in blood pressure when standing up, positive provocation manoeuvres for BPPV) may help to narrow the differential diagnosis. Higher age, multiple vascular risk factors, and an abrupt onset make a vascular cause more likely. The diagnostic work-up should include MRI and magnetic resonance angiography (MRA) searching for stenosis, diffusion restrictions, and past infarcts. Treatment options aim to prevent further TIAs or a stroke.

9.3.3 Anterior circulation stroke

Whereas acute dizziness or vertigo is reported in 50–70% in posterior circulation stroke and represents an important diagnostic feature, only 13% of patients with (mostly right-sided) ischaemic stroke in the anterior circulation suffer from dizziness. Furthermore, rotational sensations (vertigo) in anterior circulation stroke seem to be the exception. In these patients, dizziness—if observed—is typically mild and therefore not the leading finding. Consequently, other signs of stroke will usually guide the clinician to the correct diagnosis.

9.3.4 Brainstem and cerebellar haemorrhages

Intraparenchymal bleeding in the posterior fossa probably causes about 4% of all central AVS syndromes, but is potentially fatal due to possible brainstem compression and obstructive hydrocephalus. As in ischaemic stroke, signs of cerebellar or brainstem deficits will lead the clinician to the diagnosis. More frequently than in ischaemic cerebellar stroke, accompanying occipital headache or nuchal rigidity is reported. Loss of consciousness may also favour haemorrhage over stroke, as every second patient with a cerebellar bleeding experiences loss of consciousness in the first 24 hours. In cases with repetitive vomiting, other signs suggestive of beginning herniation (e.g. new gaze palsy or mydriatic non-responsive pupil followed by a decreasing level of consciousness) must be searched for. Note that vomiting (in the absence of other gastrointestinal symptoms) can be the presenting symptom, potentially being misinterpreted as acute gastroenteritis. Possible causes of brainstem or cerebellar haemorrhage (Figure 9.3) are hypertension, a ruptured arteriovenous malformation (AVM) or cavernous angioma, aneurysms or bleeding into a tumour, and head trauma. However, dizziness or vertigo may also result from supratentorial bleeding (or other space-occupying processes as oedema or rapid tumour growth) with

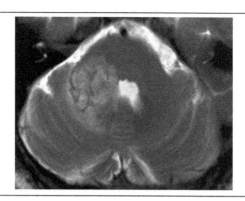

Figure 9.3 Right-sided cerebellar haemorrhage at the level of the inferior cerebellar peduncle. This 67-year-old patient presented with acute-onset parietal head-ache, followed by prolonged vertigo and severe imbalance making walking unaided impossible, numbness in the face on the right side, and uncoordinated movements of the right side. On clinical examination, an acute cerebellar syndrome with right-sided hemiataxia, slight dysarthria, gaze-evoked nystagmus, and a trigeminal sensory deficit on the right side were noted. The aetiology of the haemorrhage remained unclear, no previous history of hypertension was known, and the conventional cerebral angiography demonstrated no vascular malformations. MRI image courtesy of the Department of Neuroradiology, University Hospital Zurich, Switzerland.

subsequent herniation and brainstem compression. Depending on the volume of the bleed and signs suggestive of herniation, a neurosurgical intervention (posterior fossa craniotomy, shunting) may be lifesaving, alongside conservative care aiming for tight blood pressure control and cardiac monitoring.

9.3.5 Hemodynamic and compression syndromes

In rare circumstances, large-angle head turns may provoke posterior circulation TIA, termed **RVAS**. As a prerequisite to RVAS, vertebral blood supply provided by a single or dominant vertebral artery is assumed. In this condition, head turns contralateral to the dominant artery may lead to vertebrobasilar insufficiency by mechanical occlusion, resulting in head-position-dependent dizziness or vertigo. This syndrome is said to lead, in extreme cases, to complete infarction due to repetitive vertebral artery injury, called **bow hunter's stroke**. Possible cases of RVAS must first be assessed for carotid sinus syndrome (see Chapter 10) and horizontal canal BPPV (see Chapter 6), as these (more frequent) conditions may also be triggered by head rotation.

The vertebral arteries originate from the subclavian arteries. Proximal subclavian artery stenosis (mainly due to atherosclerosis) may result in reversal of vertebral artery blood flow as documented by duplex sonography. This, however, leads to symptomatic cerebral hypoperfusion and subsequent neurological symptoms in a minority of patients. The most frequent symptoms of this so-called '**subclavian steal syndrome**' are vertigo (61%), syncope (44%), and arm claudication (33%). Differences in arterial blood pressure between the two arms and symptoms triggered by arm exercise may provide valuable hints. Completed stroke in subclavian steal syndrome seems infrequent, and its risk is still debated.

9.3.6 Orthostatic tremor

Postural imbalance has a wide differential diagnosis (including peripheral polyneuropathy (PNP), hypotension, cerebellar degeneration, and chronic vestibular insufficiency). In a small fraction of these patients a position-dependent, high-frequency (typically 13–18 Hz) tremor restricted to the leg muscles can be found. Typically, this so-called **'orthostatic tremor'** is described by the patients as a feeling of unsteadiness and is present only while standing, but not while walking around or sitting. When orthostatic tremor is suspected, the clinician should search for this condition by holding a stethoscope to the leg muscles (as a thumping sound like a helicopter can be heard in orthostatic tremor) and order an electromyography study for confirmation. Associated neurological abnormalities are present in 25–30% of patients and mainly concern other extrapyramidal symptoms. Complaints are progressive in about 70% of cases, and response to treatment with clonazepam (considered a first-line therapy), gabapentin, or dopaminergic substances is often disappointing.

9.4 Dizziness, vertigo, and gait imbalance in MS

MS is an autoimmune disorder of the central nervous system (CNS) leading to inflammation, focal demyelination, and neurodegeneration. Whereas immune dysregulation seems to play a critical role, the aetiology of MS remains unknown. Its prevalence is around 30–110/100,000, and its incidence peaks at age 30, affecting more women than men (ratio 2–3:1). During the course of illness, up to 36% of MS patients will at some point complain of vertigo (Swingler and Compston 1992).

Acute and prolonged spontaneous vertigo along with a pathologic HIT in a patient with known MS strongly points to focal demyelination at the root entry zone of the vestibular nerve or within the vestibular nuclei (note that a gaze palsy may make interpretation of the HIT impossible). In patients with AVS, MS is the second most frequent central cause, reflecting 11% of all central-type AVS cases. Differential diagnosis includes VN, MD, or AICA stroke, with hearing impairment in the latter two diagnoses. Although a focal plaque of demyelination may lead to isolated AVS, in most cases other signs and symptoms supporting a central origin of AVS can be found. Position-dependent dizziness or vertigo along with positional nystagmus (see Section 9.7) may emerge from focal brainstem or cerebellar demyelination. However, in patients with MS, coincidental BPPV remains the most frequent cause of acute vertigo.

Gait unsteadiness is a frequent complaint in the course of MS disease progression and may emerge from combined sensory loss, ataxia, and spasticity. Visual vertigo can be found in conditions leading to double vision or blurred vision on head turns, such as internuclear ophthalmoplegia caused by lesions along the median longitudinal fascicle or acquired pendular nystagmus due to brainstem lesions. Young age, previous symptoms suggesting an inflammatory disorder as optic neuritis, and a lack of vascular risk factors may suggest MS rather than a cerebrovascular disorder. Nonetheless, the initial diagnostic approach on the ED will be identical until imaging points towards a non-vascular cause of the condition. Characteristic MRI findings in MS include T2-hyperintense lesions located in the corpus callosum and the periventricular and subcortical white matter, with a flame-like shape oriented perpendicular to the lateral ventricles on sagittal images. Acute lesions will show contrast enhancement. T1-hypointense lesions (black holes) point to past inflammatory changes with axonal loss. Besides a full work-up for suspected MS, the indication for urgent high-dose steroid treatment and for a disease-modifying therapy needs to be evaluated. If gait imbalance is a relevant issue, a treatment trial with sustained-release 4-AP may be initiated along with vestibular rehabilitation. Whereas acute vertigo will resolve in most cases, gait disturbances usually show a progressive course in MS.

9.5 Gait imbalance and dizziness related to extrapyramidal disorders

With bradykinesia, postural instability, and stiffness, extrapyramidal degenerative disorders are an important differential diagnosis in elderly patients who complain about progressive gait imbalance and (near) falls. Whereas Parkinson's disease (PD) with clear motor signs (asymmetric resting tremor, akinesia and rigidity along with postural instability) is readily recognized, it may be missed in early stages, when symptom onset is insidious, motor symptoms are subtle, and non-motor symptoms (olfactory dysfunction, sleep disturbances, erectile dysfunction, anxiety, impaired executive functions, orthostatic hypotension) are not linked to Parkinson's disorders. Searching for poverty and slowness of movements, subtle differences in muscle tone (as may also be noticed when applying the HIT), and asking for non-motor symptoms, especially olfactory deficits, constipation, and rapid eye movement (REM)-sleep behaviour disorders (RBD) will help the clinician to identify patients with imbalance and falls related to extrapyramidal degenerative disorders (see differential diagnosis of falls in Chapter 11 for more details).

9.6 Gait imbalance and dizziness related to ataxia

Ataxia, which describes a lack of coordination of movements, represents a heterogeneous group of disorders with varying onset (acute, subacute, insidious) and disease course (remitting, stable, progressive). Whereas hereditary ataxia (see Section 9.5.2) may become manifest during childhood or early adulthood, patients with adult-onset progressive ataxia typically have a negative family history regarding gait problems (Klockgether 2010). In these patients, the entire spectrum of causes for ataxia must be considered.

Depending on the aetiology of ataxia, patients may instead present with a cerebellar syndrome or sensory loss. Cerebellar syndromes lead to an incoordination of movements in general and may therefore affect numerous systems to varying extent, including gait (wide-based, ataxic steps), posture (increased sway), extremity movements (dysmetric and with intention tremor when approaching the target), swallowing, speech, and eye movements (dysmetric saccades, saccadic smooth pursuit, gravity-dependent downbeat nystagmus). **These patients typically do not report episodic vertigo or dizziness, with the exception of patients with SCA6 or EA type 1-6**. If ataxia is related to an afferent deficit, the most prominent findings will be those of sensory loss, which may be accompanied by spasticity (pointing to a spinal cord problem) or lack of tendon reflexes (pointing to PNP). Identifying such symptoms, but also searching for extrapyramidal movement disorders, other pyramidal tract signs, and cortical disturbances is important in the differential diagnosis of ataxia. Specific information about the rate of disease progression, alcohol intake, exposure to toxins, concomitant medical conditions (chronic infections, cancer), symptoms suggestive of cancer or autonomic dysfunction (orthostatic hypotension, decreased sweating, erectile dysfunction, urinary retention) should be obtained. If the diagnostic work-up does not reveal an acquired or hereditary cause of ataxia, a diagnosis of sporadic adult-onset ataxia (SAOA) of unknown origin will be made. Treatment is often symptomatic only and aims to secure swallowing, preserve ambulation, and prevent falls. Regular follow-up visits are essential, as initially additional signs such as orthostatic dysfunction (pointing to ataxia secondary to MSA) may be absent.

9.6.1 Sporadic and acquired ataxias

Acute-onset cerebellar ataxia may be linked to acute alcohol or drug (phenytoin, lithium, carbamazepine) intoxication and typically resolves after removal of the causing agent. Infectious/parainfectious disorders, cerebellar stroke, or haemorrhage and WE are other conditions leading to acute cerebellar ataxia. Ataxia related to immune-mediated (paraneoplastic) inflammation or infections, such as sporadic CJD (sCJD), may present subacutely. Amongst the causes of slowly progressive acquired ataxia, alcoholic cerebellar degeneration (ACD) is probably the most frequent. Slowly progressive sporadic ataxia may also be linked to MSA-cerebellar type (MSA-C), severe polyneuropathy, or posterior cord spinal lesions (with the latter two leading to profound sensory ataxia). Acute sensory ataxia may result from Guillain-Barré syndrome and Miller-Fisher syndrome and may persist in chronic inflammatory demyelinating polyneuropathy (CIDP).

9.6.1.1 Toxic cerebellar degeneration

Besides ACD, progressive cerebellar loss may be associated with other substances, including various drugs (lithium, phenytoin, amiodarone; usually with long-term exposure), chemotherapeutics (5-fluorouracil, cytosine arabinoside), and heavy metal poisoning. Chronic alcohol abuse may cause profound cerebellar degeneration via both direct toxicity and vitamin B_1 deficiency, clinically presenting as severe ataxia of the lower extremities and gait ataxia, which may progress substantially within weeks to a few months. Characteristically, the arms and eye movements and speech are relatively spared. ACD seems to be one of the most frequent causes of chronic cerebellar ataxia (Klockgether 2010) and may be present in up to 27% of chronic alcohol users. On MRI, vermal atrophy can be found. Immediate interruption of the exposure to these substances (including alcohol intake) is essential for the prognosis. As a preventive measure, vitamin B_1 supplementation in chronic alcohol users and during chemotherapy including 5-fluorouracil or cytosine arabinoside is recommended. If ataxia is evolving rapidly and accompanied by other symptoms, such as double vision, neuropathy, seizures, and mental confusion, WE is an important differential diagnosis, mandating rapid supplementation with vitamin B_1.

9.6.1.2 Immune-mediated cerebellar degeneration, including paraneoplastic syndromes

Immune-mediated cerebellar degeneration may be associated with a variety of disorders, amongst which paraneoplastic syndromes are of special importance due to their association with (yet undiagnosed) cancer. Other immune-mediated disorders leading to ataxia include anti-glutamic acid decarboxylase (GAD) ataxia in insulin-dependent diabetes, ataxia in asymptomatic celiac disease (although this entity is controversial), and steroid-responsive encephalopathy associated with autoimmune thyroiditis (SREAT, previously called Hashimoto encephalopathy). For subacute progressive ataxia, therefore, checking glucose levels, thyroid function, and evaluating for celiac disease may be of diagnostic relevance.

A paraneoplastic cerebellar degeneration must be considered if the course of ataxia is rapidly progressive within few months, as immune-mediated cerebellar degeneration may precede cancer (small-cell lung cancer, ovarian and breast cancer, Hodgkin's lymphoma) by months to years. The diagnostic approach includes searching for antibodies with known association to cerebellar ataxia (including anti-Yo, anti-Tr, anti-mGluR1, anti-CV2, anti-VGCC, and anti-Ri), and the MRI is initially often normal. Of priority is a thorough and—if negative—repetitive search for a primary tumour. The paraneoplastic syndrome (with few exceptions as in Hodgkin's lymphoma) usually does not improve when treating the underlying cancer or upon immunosuppression.

Fluctuating rigidity, muscle stiffness with superimposed unpredictable painful muscle spasms, lumbar hyperlordosis, and frequent falls are characteristic findings of stiff person syndrome (SPS) (see Hadavi et al 2011 for review). SPS is a rare autoimmune disorder (prevalence 1–2/1,000,000) associated with GAD-antibodies in 60–80% of cases, whereas about 5% of cases have a paraneoplastic aetiology. The pathophysiological correlate to the stiffness is continuous motor unit activity on electromyography. In the differential diagnosis, patients with gait imbalance, falls, and painful muscle stiffness should turn the clinician's attention to possible SPS. SPS is associated with other autoimmune disorders such as type 1 diabetes (35%), epilepsy (10%), and cerebellar ataxia (10%), the presence of which may further support a diagnosis of SPS. Treatment aims to reduce spasms by use of gamma-aminobutyric acid (GABA)-ergic substances as diazepam and to suppress the immune system by use of immunomodulatory substances such as intravenous immunoglobulins.

9.6.1.3 Acquired vitamin deficiency

Reduced levels of vitamins B_1, B_{12}, and E, possibly related to dietary restrictions, chronic vomiting and malabsorption, may lead to acquired ataxia. Evaluating for other signs of vitamin B_1 (see Section 9.6.1 regarding WE), B_{12} (polyneuropathy or myelopathy leading to sensory ataxia, macrocytic anaemia), and E (gastrointestinal disorders, other cerebellar signs, sensory neuropathy) deficiency is essential in the differential diagnosis. If the blood work-up confirms insufficient levels of one of these vitamins, appropriate supplementation is mandatory in addition to treating the underlying cause (if identified). Note that vitamin E deficiency can also be hereditary; however, in that case it usually presents at age 20 or before.

9.6.1.4 Ataxia related to CNS infections

Cerebellar ataxia may be secondary to acute viral infections (e.g. varicella and infectious mononucleosis) or related to chronic CNS infections and may be accompanied by vertigo and dizziness. Onset of complaints is typically abrupt if related to acute viral infections. Recovery from post-viral acute ataxia is usually achieved within few weeks. Chronic CNS infections, on the other hand, may lead to ataxia that slowly progresses over time, possibly accompanied by dizziness. In neurosyphilis (resulting in damage of the posterior spinal columns), ataxia is of sensory origin and signs of cerebellar dysfunction are therefore lacking. Whipple's disease, a systemic infection caused by *Tropheryma whipplei*, is characterized by cerebellar ataxia accompanied by fever, arthritis, and gastrointestinal problems (diarrhoea, abdominal pain). If CNS infection is suspected, the patient should be screened for HIV infection, as this broadens the differential diagnosis considerably, including various opportunistic infections and primary CNS lymphoma. The combination of rapidly progressive cerebellar ataxia and steep decline in cognitive functions is a red flag and must raise the suspicion for the cerebellar (ataxic) variant of sCJD. Increased 14-3-3 protein in cerebrospinal fluid (CSF) and characteristic MRI findings (cortical ribboning and basal ganglia signal changes on DWI and fluid-attenuated inversion recovery (FLAIR) sequences) may further support this diagnosis, whereas characteristic electroencephalogram (EEG) findings are typically lacking in the ataxic variant. In addition, the clinician should consider SREAT, WE, and paraneoplastic cerebellar disease.

9.6.1.5 Other acquired or sporadic causes

Superficial siderosis. Repeated subarachnoidal bleeding related to vascular abnormalities or tumours or secondary to neurosurgical procedures leads to the accumulation of haemoglobin and free iron on the surface of the brain and spinal cord. Subsequently, damage to cerebellar structures, cranial nerves, and the spinal cord may result. Patients with superficial siderosis may complain of hearing loss and may present with pyramidal signs along with progressive cerebellar ataxia (Figure 9.4). Key to the correct diagnosis is the demonstration of linear T2-hypointensities on the surface of the brain and the spinal cord along with xanthochromasia in the CSF. Removal of the source of bleeding may stop further progression.

Structural disorders. Congenital Arnold-Chiari malformations with caudal displacement of deformed cerebellar tonsils (paraflocculi), cerebellar neoplasms (primary or metastases), and traumatic brain injury including the cerebellum may lead to acute or episodic cerebellar ataxia and CPV (see 9.8). The diagnosis is readily made on sagittal MRI sequences (Figure 9.5), although more subtle tonsillar herniation related to Chiari malformation, cerebellar tumours, or lumboperitoneal CSF shunts may be missed on imaging. Normal pressure hydrocephalus (NPH) should be considered if ataxic gait is accompanied by cognitive decline and urinary incontinence. Enlarged ventricles on computed tomography (CT) or MRI images with little or no cortical atrophy and improvement after large volume (30–40 ml) spinal taps further support a diagnosis of NPH. In these patients, the benefits and downsides (shunt infections, overdrainage leading to subdural hematoma) of ventriculo-peritoneal shunting need to be addressed before applying this procedure.

9.6.2 Hereditary cerebellar ataxias

A positive family history for gait disturbances and early symptom onset may favour a hereditary ataxia; however, lack of familial clustering and adult-onset of complaints does not rule out a genetic background. Therefore, in adult-onset ataxia, a hereditary form also has to be taken into account. This has been observed for Friedreich's ataxia

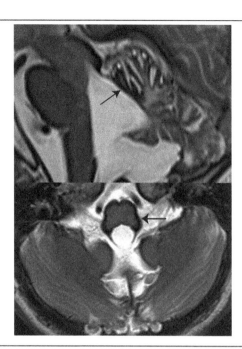

Figure 9.4 Superficial siderosis in a patient with progressive cerebellar (gait ataxia, gaze-evoked nystagmus) and pyramidal signs and hearing loss. On MRI, extensive haemosiderin deposits (in black, indicated by the arrows) on the surface of the brainstem and the cerebellum including the superior vermis (top view) are accompanied by severe atrophy of vestibulo-cerebellar structures including the nodulus, superior vermis, and the flocculus as well as enlargement of the fourth ventricle. MRI image courtesy of the Department of Neuroradiology, University Hospital Zurich, Switzerland.

(FRDA; symptom onset after age 25 in 15% of cases) and lysosomal storage disorders such as Niemann-Pick disease or ataxia telangiectasia, all belonging to the group of autosomal-recessive ataxias (for an extensive review, see Fogel and Perlman 2007). However, most autosomal-recessive ataxias become symptomatic before age 20.

SCAs (estimated prevalence: 1–3/100,000) and hereditary EAs belong to the autosomal-dominant cerebellar ataxias. SCAs present with abnormalities of both the spinal cord and the cerebellum and may be the underlying cause of adult-onset ataxia without obvious clues pointing to a hereditary form in 2–22% of cases (Klockgether 2010). Currently, over 30 SCAs are known. Based on their pathophysiology, they can be divided in three subgroups: polyglutamine expansion disorders (SCA1, SCA2, SCA3, SCA7, SCA17, and dentatorubral-pallidoluysian atrophy (DRPLA)) being prone to genetic anticipation (younger age of onset and increased severity in successive generations) and inverse correlation between age of onset and the length of the repeat; channelopathies (SCA6, EA1, EA2); and gene expression disorders (repeat expansions outside of coding regions; SCA8, SCA10, and SCA12). Accompanying signs (eye movement abnormalities, seizures, movement disorders, pyramidal tract lesions, visual loss,

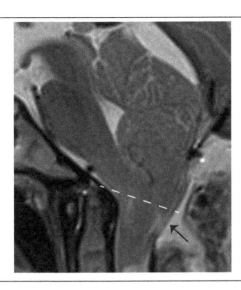

Figure 9.5 Arnold-Chiari malformation type 1. This 16-year-old patient presented with episodic vertigo and progressive gait ataxia. Sagittal MRI shows elongated and caudally displaced cerebellar tonsils (indicated by the black arrow), with the tips of the tonsils about 13 mm (normal range: < 3 mm) below the foramen magnum (indicated by the dashed white line). MRI image courtesy of the Department of Neuroradiology, University Hospital Zurich, Switzerland.

and polyneuropathy) may help in identifying different types of SCAs, whereas SCA6 may present as a pure cerebellar syndrome. SCA1, SCA2, and SCA3 are responsible for 40–80% (depending on regional differences in prevalence due to founder effects) of all SCAs. Eye movement abnormalities include very slow saccades (SCA2), hypometric saccades and gaze-evoked nystagmus (SCA3), downbeat nystagmus, periodic alternating nystagmus, and gaze-evoked nystagmus (SCA6), and bilateral vestibulopathy (SCA1 and SCA3). The most frequent of the SCAs observed with late onset is SCA6, linked to a mutation in the P/Q-type voltage-gated calcium channel (in the CACNA1A gene). MRI in SCAs may be helpful in identifying the extent of cerebellar atrophy. However, to determine the subtype of SCA, genetic testing (if the gene mutation is known) is required.

Transient ataxia and associated cerebellar signs of variable duration are the hallmarks of EAs and are typically triggered by stress or exercise. Whereas in EA2 (the most frequent form) spells last hours to days, in EA1 the spells usually last only seconds to minutes. In the interval, findings may be discrete or non-detectable. EA2 is caused by a mutation in the CACNA1A gene that encodes a subunit for voltage-gated calcium-channels and may be associated with epilepsy and migraine.

X-linked ataxias, such as fragile-X tremor ataxia syndrome (FXTAS), may also lead to ataxia. FXTAS is a trinucleotide expansion disorder and should be considered if progressive adult-onset ataxia emerges in the context of profound tremor. On examination, parkinsonian features, neuropathy, and cognitive deficits may be observed. Whereas MRI may reveal characteristic signal changes (e.g. within the middle cerebellar peduncles) combined with diffuse brain atrophy, the diagnosis is confirmed by genetic testing (e.g. *FMR1* mutation). Progressive cerebellar ataxia with adult-onset combined with neuromuscular complaints (early fatigue on exercise) may point towards an underlying mitochondrial disorder. Muscle biopsy in these patients may show characteristic changes (e.g. ragged-red fibres and cyclooxygenase (COX)-deficient fibres); however, genetic testing of the mitochondrial DNA is required to confirm the diagnosis.

Hereditary cerebellar ataxias typically show a slowly progressive course, and there are no targeted treatment options to delay or even stop their evolvement. Vestibular physiotherapy, aids for preventing falls, and treating disorders related to the ataxia (as, for example, seizures in EA2) should be considered. Channelopathies such as SCA6 and EA2 may benefit from treatment with acetazolamide or 4-AP, a voltage-gated potassium channel blocker that restores the severely diminished precision of pacemaking in Purkinje cells and increases the inhibitory drive of Purkinje cells. Potential benefits from 4-AP include a reduction in downbeat nystagmus and in gait ataxia, but contraindications such as known cardiac arrhythmia and epilepsy need to be considered. A treatment trial with 4-AP should also be performed in suitable patients with SAOA.

9.6.3 Sporadic degenerative ataxias

SAOA is considered a diagnostic challenge (Figure 9.6), and an obvious acquired or hereditary cause is often lacking. In these cases, disorders with sporadic cerebellar

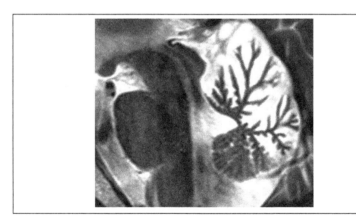

Figure 9.6 Presumed hereditary adult-onset ataxia. This 47-year-old patient has a history of progressive gait imbalance, dysarthria, and oscillopsia. On clinical examination, cerebellar ataxia (gait, limbs) and ocular motor disturbances (slight downbeat nystagmus, moderate gaze-evoked nystagmus, saccadic smooth pursuit, bilaterally deficient HIT) were noted. On MRI, marked cerebellar atrophy, predominantly of the superior vermis and the cerebellar hemispheres, is demonstrated. Based on the positive family history (mother and one brother with similar symptoms), a hereditary autosomal-dominant ataxia is suspected, although genetic testing for FXTAS, DRPLA, and SCA1, SCA2, SCA3, SCA6, SCA7, SCA10, SCA12, and SCA17 was negative. MRI image courtesy of the Medizinisch Radiologisches Institut, Zurich, Switzerland.

Table 9.4 Predictive factors in the differential diagnosis of SAOA (modified after Klockgether 2010)

Predictor	Associated disorders	Diagnostic hallmarks
Chronic alcohol intake, exposure to heavy metals, drugs (AED, ChT)[†]	ACD, toxic cerebellar degeneration	Lab: ACD (elevated liver enzymes, macro-cytosis), toxic (heavy metals) MRI: ACD (vermal atrophy)
Autonomic failure	MSA-C, HSAN,[†] diabetic neuropathy	MRI: MSA-C (hot cross bun sign, pontine and cerebellar atrophy) ENMG: HSAN,[†] diabetic PNP
Rapid progression	sCJD, WE, post-viral immune-mediated ataxia, SREAT, stroke or haemorrhage	MRI: sCJD (FLAIR and DWI: cortical ribboning, hyperintensities in basal ganglia, thalamus, pulvinar), WE (signal changes in medial thalamus, mamillary bodies, around 3rd ventricle), stroke/ haemorrhage lab: WE (B_1 deficiency), sCJD (14-3-3 protein in CSF)
Malignant disorders	PCD,[†] cerebellar metastasis	Anti-neuronal antibodies: PCD[†]
CNS infection or inflammation	HIV, neurosyphilis, SREAT, sCJD	Serology: HIV, neuro-syphilis TPO[†]-antibodies, rapid response to steroids: SREAT
Gastrointestinal complaints (diarrhoea)	Whipple's disease, Vitamin E deficiency, celiac disease	PAS[†]-positive staining and PCR: Whipple's disease. Serology: celiac disease
Sensory ataxia	PNP (B_{12}-deficit, CIDP, diabetic), FRDA, myelopathy (syphilis)	Lab: B_{12} (HTC,[†] B_{12} level) ENMG[‡]: CIDP, B_{12}, diabetic PNP Serology: neuro-syphilis Genetic testing: FRDA[†]

[†] Abbreviations: AED: anti-epileptic drugs; ChT: chemotherapy; ENMG: electroneuromyography; HSAN: hereditary sensory autonomic neuropathy; HTC: holotranscobalamin; PAS: periodic acid-Schiff; PCD: paraneoplastic cerebellar degeneration; TPO: thyroid peroxidase.

degeneration have to be considered, including MSA-C (see Table 9.4). A progressive cerebellar syndrome with ataxia, dysarthria, and ocular motor disturbances accompanied by severe autonomic dysfunction (orthostatic hypotension, urinary and respiratory dysfunction, and RBD) and (less prominent in the cerebellar variant) parkinsonian features that respond poorly to levodopa should raise suspicion for MSA-C, which belongs to the alpha-synucleinopathies. Average age of onset is around 55 years. With regards to the autonomic dysfunction (first symptom in up to 40% of MSA-C patients), severe (diabetic) autonomic polyneuropathy is a differential diagnosis for orthostatic hypotension; however, in these cases, ataxia will be sensory and cerebellar (and parkinsonian) signs will be missing. There is no specific treatment, and a patient with MSA-C experiences a progressive loss of mobility, requiring a wheelchair after four to five years. In patients with SAOA, orthostatic hypotension (i.e. drop in systolic (≥ 30 mmHg) or diastolic (≥ 15 mmHg) blood pressure after three minutes of standing), frequent falls, RBD, and parkinsonian features are red flags and should reinforce the search for MSA-C, including brain MRI (search for atrophy of putamen, middle cerebellar peduncle, pons, or cerebellum, and pontocerebellar signal hyperintensities).

SAOA with unknown origin often starts around age 50 and is considered to be one of the most frequent types of ataxia (prevalence 7–8/100,000). It has a considerably more benign (but still progressive) course than, for example, MSA-C, with unaided walking preserved 12 years after symptom onset in half of patients (Klockgether 2010). Whereas imaging usually demonstrates degeneration restricted to the cerebellum, subtle non-cerebellar signs may be found on clinical examination, including sensory disturbances and pyramidal tract defects.

9.7 **Epileptic vertigo and dizziness**

Dizziness and vertigo are frequent aura symptoms, preceding epileptic seizures in up to 70% of cases. Specifically, rotatory vertigo is mentioned by 6–19% of patients with temporal, parietal, and occipital lobe seizures or generalized epilepsy. Obviously, in patients treated with anticonvulsant drugs, medication side effects or unrelated vestibular disorders may explain these complaints in a considerable number of cases. Nonetheless, in probably less than 1% of all new cases of epilepsy, true isolated epileptic vertigo or dizziness may mimic vestibular disorders by activation of parieto-temporal (vestibular-related) areas. These episodes typically last seconds only. Most patients with epileptic dizziness or vertigo will have other clinical features of epilepsy, such as additional aura symptoms, absences, or generalized convulsions. Nausea reported in the recovery phase after epileptic seizures or nystagmus observed during the spells may further complicate the distinction from vestibular disorders. Due to their brief duration and spontaneous occurrence, the differential diagnosis focuses on VM and vestibular paroxysmia (VP). As a first step, the clinician should ask about symptoms specific for epilepsy, although video-electroencephalographic telemetry and brain MRI may eventually be required to reliably exclude seizures as a cause for recurrent, brief, and spontaneous dizziness or vertigo.

9.8 **Central positional vertigo (CPV)**

Positional nystagmus is the hallmark of peripheral BPPV (see Chapter 6), presenting with a characteristic pattern, including a latency of a few seconds and duration of 5–20 seconds. However, position-dependent nystagmus may also be related to central pathologies, making it difficult to distinguish between central and peripheral BPPV. It is not possible to differentiate between the two from the results of positional physical examination (latency, fatigability etc.; Büttner et al 1999).

For the clinician, red flags in the patient with presumed BPPV are atypical presentation of nystagmus (such as purely upbeat, downbeat, or pure torsional nystagmus), lack of vertigo/dizziness in the presence of positional nystagmus, and subtle central (cerebellar ocular motor or brainstem) signs. Although BPPV of central origin is rare in comparison to the peripheral one, one may only be more or less relaxed and suppose a peripheral origin in very typical cases of posterior canalolithiasis (see Chapter 6) which can easily be improved by one or two reposition manoeuvres.

Otherwise, it is better to be on the safe side by ordering a brain MRI and searching for a central cause. Demyelinating, ischaemic or haemorrhagic lesions located in the cerebellum (superior cerebellar peduncle, dorsal vermis, or nodulus) or dorsolateral to the fourth ventricle may lead to CPV as well as MSA-C, craniocervical anomalies, and tumours of the fourth ventricle.

References and Further Reading

Büttner U., Helmchen C., Brandt T. (1999) Diagnostic criteria for central versus peripheral positioning nystagmus and vertigo: a review. *Acta Otolaryngol.* **119**, 1–5.

Edlow J. A., Newman-Toker D. E., Savitz S.I. (2008) Diagnosis and initial management of cerebellar infarction. *Lancet Neurol.* **7**, 951–64.

Eggers S. D. (2007) Migraine-related vertigo: diagnosis and treatment. *Curr Pain Headache Rep.* **11**, 217–26.

Fogel B. L. and Perlman S. (2007) Clinical features and molecular genetics of autosomal recessive cerebellar ataxias. *Lancet Neurol.* **6**, 245–57.

Goadsby P. J. and Sprenger T. (2010) Current practice and future directions in the prevention and acute management of migraine. *Lancet Neurol.* **9**, 285–98.

Gottesman R. F., Sharma P., Robinson K. A. *et al.* (2012) Clinical characteristics of symptomatic vertebral artery dissection: a systematic review. *Neurologist.* **18**, 245–54.

Hadavi S., Noyce A. J., Leslie R. D. *et al.* (2011) Stiff person syndrome. *Pract Neurol.* **11**, 272–82.

Hwang D. Y., Silva G. S., Furie K. L. *et al.* (2012) Comparative sensitivity of computed tomography vs. magnetic resonance imaging for detecting acute posterior fossa infarct. *J Emerg Med.* **42**, 559–65.

International Headache Society Classification Subcommittee (2004) International classification of headache disorders. 2nd edn. *Cephalalgia.* **24** (Suppl 1), 1–160.

Ishiyama G. and Ishiyama A. (2011) Vertebrobasilar infarcts and ischemia. *Otolaryngol Clin North Am.* **44**, 415–35.

Klockgether T. (2010) Sporadic ataxia with adult onset: classification and diagnostic criteria. *Lancet Neurol.* **9**, 94–104.

Lee H. (2009) Neuro-otological aspects of cerebellar stroke syndrome. *J Clin Neurol.* **5**, 65–73.

Neuhauser H. and Lempert T. (2009) Vestibular migraine. *Neurol Clin.* **27**, 379–91.

Silberstein S. D., Holland S., Freitag F. *et al.* (2012) Evidence-based guideline update: pharmacologic treatment for episodic migraine prevention in adults: report of the Quality Standards Subcommittee of the American Academy of Neurology and the American Headache Society. *Neurology.* **78**, 1337–45.

Swingler R. J. and Compston D. A. (1992) The morbidity of multiple sclerosis. *Q J Med.* **83**, 325–37.

Tarnutzer A. A., Berkowitz A. L., Robinson K. A. *et al.* (2011) Does my dizzy patient have a stroke? A systematic review of bedside diagnosis in acute vestibular syndrome. *CMAJ.* **183**, E571–92.

118

Chapter 10

Medical, non-vestibular causes of dizziness or vertigo

Key points

- Approximately 50% of patients presenting with dizziness or vertigo to the emergency department (ED) have an underlying non-vestibular medical disorder, whereas only about 33% are diagnosed with a neurotological (vestibular) disease.
- The percentage of dangerous disorders in dizzy patients presenting to the emergency room increases with age (from <10% at age ≤25 to >25% at age ≥ 75 years).
- Dizziness and vertigo have a broad differential diagnosis. Thus, signs and symptoms atypical for an underlying vestibular disorder combined with a normal neurotological examination mandate a more extensive evaluation.
- Frequent non-vestibular causes include vasovagal syncope and dangerous conditions such as cardiac arrhythmia, electrolyte or fluid disturbances, cardiovascular disorders, anaemia secondary to gastrointestinal bleeding, and hypoglycaemia.

10.1 Introduction

New onset dizziness or vertigo has a broad differential diagnosis distributed across many medical fields, forcing the clinician to keep the focus of potential underlying disorders wide. This includes fields in which the individual clinician may feel uncertain or lacks experience. Consecutively, he/she may diagnose conditions that fall into the field of one's expertise too frequently, which may result in delayed and inadequate treatment with potentially devastating consequences, for example, when vertigo secondary to cardiac arrhythmia remains undiagnosed. After having discussed many conditions related to the vestibular field in the previous chapters, we encourage the reader to think across specialties when dealing with dizzy patients. In the following, we discuss selected non-vestibular medical conditions linked to dizziness or vertigo based on their frequency and hazardousness.

10.2 **Aetiology of dizziness or vertigo unrelated to vestibular disorders**

In a representative sample of ED visits with a presenting complaint of dizziness or vertigo, Newman-Toker and colleagues found that otologic/vestibular disorders make up only about 33% of diagnoses, whereas non-vestibular, general medical conditions were more frequent (about 50%) (Newman-Toker et al 2008). Categories provided by most studies segregating the underlying cause of dizziness or vertigo in patients presenting to the ED were oto-vestibular (13–34%), other neurological disorders (5–11%), cardiovascular disorders including cardiac arrhythmia (4–21%), psychiatric diagnoses (2–14%), and non-cardiovascular general medical diagnoses (8–28%). The five most frequent non-vestibular causes according to Newman-Toker and colleagues (2008) were vasovagal syncope (6.6%), electrolyte and fluid disorders (5.6%), cardiac arrhythmia (3.2%), anaemia (1.6%), and hypoglycaemia (1.4%). Whereas some of these disorders are recurrent and benign, others are potentially life threatening if not recognized rapidly (see Table 10.1).

10.3 **When to think about non-vestibular causes of dizziness or vertigo**

In otological disorders, the clinical examination will demonstrate signs related to disturbances of the peripheral and central audio-vestibular system, including nystagmus

Table 10.1 Benign and potentially dangerous non-vestibular causes of dizziness or vertigo

Benign, self-limiting disorders	Dangerous, potentially life-threatening disorders
Circulation • Vasovagal (pre)syncope • Carotid sinus syndrome • Orthostatic hypotension • Postural orthostatic tachycardia syndrome (POTS)	Circulation • Fluid and electrolyte disorders (e.g. hyponatraemia) • Anaemia, e.g. due to gastrointestinal bleeding • Aortic dissection, ruptured aortic aneurysm • Pulmonary embolism • Insufficiently treated hypertension
Psychiatric disorders • Anxiety and panic disorders • Depression • Chronic mild hyperventilation	Cardiac disorders • Cardiac arrhythmia • Angina pectoris • Myocardial infarction
Metabolic/toxic • Alcohol intoxication • Drug-related side effects (e.g. antihypertensive medication, diuretics, antidepressants, vasodilators) • Adverse drug reactions • Iron deficiency leading to anaemia	Metabolic/toxic • Hypoglycaemia • Drug intoxication (e.g. phenytoin, lithium, benzodiazepines) • Carbon monoxide poisoning • Alcohol withdrawal • Endocrine disorders (e.g. adrenal insufficiency)
Others • Deconditioning • Visual impairment	Others • Acute infections (e.g. pneumonia)

(spontaneous, position-dependent paroxysmal nystagmus as in benign paroxysmal positional vertigo (BPPV) or gaze-evoked), skew deviation, pathological head impulse test (HIT), hearing loss, focal neurological signs including cerebellar impairment, limb paresis, and Horner syndrome. However, acute prolonged dizziness or vertigo may present in isolation; hence only subtle ocular motor signs (HINTS (**H**ead **I**mpulse test, searching for direction-changing **N**ystagmus, and **T**est of **S**kew deviation) to INFARCT (**I**mpulse **N**ormal or **F**ast-phase **A**lternating or **R**efixation on **C**over **T**est), see Chapter 2) may be observed with obvious focal neurological findings being absent in about 50% of patients. These are the vestibular cases, which must not be missed, as they may originate from vertebrobasilar ischaemia or cerebellar haemorrhage. If the neurotological examination is inconclusive or negative in an acutely dizzy patient, non-vestibular causes have to be considered and excluded before only a symptom-related diagnosis is made and the patient is discharged. Of note, focal neurological (cerebellar) signs (including gaze-evoked nystagmus, ataxia and dysarthria) may also be secondary to systemic disorders such as drug-related neurotoxicity.

Provocation or exacerbation of complaints upon the patient standing up points towards a possible diagnosis of orthostatic hypotension and should be followed by blood pressure and heart rate measurements before and immediately after standing. A significant drop in blood pressure (>20 mmHg systolic or >10 mmHg diastolic) within three minutes is diagnostic. Orthostatic hypotension may be secondary to hypovolemia, anaemia (e.g. due to occult gastrointestinal bleeding or iron deficiency), autonomic failure (e.g. in diabetic autonomic neuropathy, neurodegenerative disorders, i.e. multiple systems atrophy(MSA)) or drug-related side effects. Complete blood count and iron levels will help identify orthostasis related to anaemia. Dizziness and vertigo are amongst the more frequent side effects of various drugs, including antihypertensive drugs, neuroleptics, barbiturates, and diuretics. Drug intoxication with neuromodulatory substances, especially antiepileptic (e.g. phenytoin, carbamazepine) and sedative drugs may lead to acute prolonged vertigo or dizziness, mandating a reduction of the dosage or a switch to a different substance in case of ongoing intolerance or drug-interactions. A drug history, especially searching for changes in drug dosage and newly prescribed drugs, is therefore mandatory in the acutely dizzy patient.

An increase in heart rate with blood pressure remaining stable during the dizzy spell (usually triggered by standing up) may point towards POTS. Vasovagal (pre)syncope typically occurs in the young and in the context of ongoing pain or fear, heat, dehydration, or prolonged standing. Prodromal symptoms are prominent and usually last seconds to minutes. They include dizziness or vertigo, diaphoresis, pallor, chest pain, dyspnoea, palpitations, and nausea.

Cardiac arrhythmia (e.g. complete heart block, ventricular tachycardia) may not only present with either dizziness or vertigo, but may lead to a transient loss of consciousness ('cardiogenic syncope') and may be misinterpreted as seizure in such situations. Age over 45 years, known heart disease, male gender, and relatively short illness duration (typically less than one year) all increase the risk for cardiac arrhythmia, but congenital structural heart diseases or innate arrhythmia may lead to cardiogenic dizziness and syncope in the young. Short dizziness spells lasting for seconds and lacking prodromal symptoms, absence of triggers, and prolonged loss of consciousness (more than two minutes) make a cardiogenic origin more likely and mandate urgent referral to a cardiologist for further diagnostic testing. Dizziness and focal neurological symptoms (Horner syndrome, stroke due to extension of dissection into the carotid arteries or secondary to decreased carotid blood flow) preceded by sudden sharp chest or back pain should raise suspicion for a possible aortic dissection.

Persistent mild hyperventilation may lead to chronic dizziness secondary to increased blood pH levels and should be considered if symptoms are clearly reduced or even disappear during physical activities and distraction. Panic and anxiety disorders may result in dizziness or vertigo but often also lead to falls and apparent loss of consciousness. Unexplained medical symptoms in the patient history, a positive psychiatric history, and a history of traumatic experiences during childhood are conditions that may point towards an underlying psychiatric disorder. Dizziness or vertigo related to a mental (e.g. panic, phobic, anxiety, depression, dissociative, somatoform) disorder may develop subsequently to an organic vestibular disorder (in about 30% of patients) or may emerge without such a condition. If identified, treatment should include behavioural therapy.

Endocrine disorders such as adrenal insufficiency may lead to changes in the fluid and electrolyte balance, whereas insulin overdosage in insulin-dependent diabetes and insulinoma are linked to hypoglycaemia. Patients that have been immobilized—usually because of critical illnesses—may complain of dizziness or vertigo along with other symptoms such as fatigue and tachycardia when mobilized again, with first symptoms typically occurring during stationary rehabilitation. Cardiovascular deconditioning may be a potential cause in such patients; however, especially in patients that have suffered systemic and severe infections, ototoxic drugs (most frequently aminoglycosides) leading to chronic vestibular insufficiency (see Chapter 7) must also be considered (see Table 10.2).

Table 10.2 Red flags for dangerous non-vestibular dizziness or vertigo	
Symptoms and signs	Potentially dangerous non-vestibular disorders
Anaemia and tachycardia	Occult bleeding, e.g. gastrointestinal, iron deficiency
Thoracic or abdominal pain	Angina pectoris, myocardial infarction, aortic dissection, ruptured aortic aneurysm
Dyspnoea	Pulmonary embolism, angina pectoris, myocardial infarction, pneumonia
Sudden transient loss of consciousness	Cardiac arrhythmia, vasovagal syncope, carotid sinus syndrome
History of diabetes mellitus	Hypoglycaemia, orthostatic hypotension (autonomic failure)
New onset medication, change in dosage of established medication	Adverse drug reactions, drug-related side effects, drug intoxication
Hypertension	Drug-related orthostatic hypotension, hypertensive encephalopathy in case of insufficient antihypertensive treatment or hypertensive crisis.
Triggers • Head turn, wearing collar or tie • Position dependency: symptoms only while standing	Associated disorder • Carotid sinus syndrome • Orthostatic hypotension, occult bleeding
Systemic inflammatory signs as fever, elevated C-reactive protein (CRP)	Infection, sepsis

10.4 Treatment of non-vestibular dizziness or vertigo and prognosis

Whereas (pre)syncope in general is considered a benign disorder, the mortality rate in cardiogenic syncope reaches 30% in the first year, underlining the need to better identify non-vestibular causes of dizziness or vertigo and initiate appropriate treatment. Reduction or cessation of drugs inducing the patient's complaints, administration of electrolyte supplements, and antiarrhythmic treatment (e.g. by medication or by placing a pacemaker/implantable conversion device) may be required—if an underlying cause can be identified at all. Treatment options for vasovagal syncope are usually non-pharmacological and emphasize avoidance of triggers and mechanical or behavioural strategies to decrease underlying orthostasis. Venous pooling can be counteracted by anti-orthostatic manoeuvres such as squatting or standing with the legs crossed.

References and Further Reading

Newman-Toker D. E., Hsieh Y. H., Camargo C. A. Jr et al. (2008) Spectrum of dizziness visits to US emergency departments: cross-sectional analysis from a nationally representative sample. *Mayo Clin Proc.* **83**, 765–75.

Chapter 11

Diagnosis of falls, dizziness in children and elderly

Key points

- Most falls are related to obvious causes (e.g. tripping over obstacles).
- Unexplained falls may occur due to vestibular (e.g. Menière's disease (MD)) or vascular causes, or because of impaired gait, such as in Parkinson's disease (PD).
- Management of falls is often symptomatic, including a structured fall risk assessment, balance training, and an evaluation for walking aids.
- Frequent causes of vertigo or dizziness in children and adolescents are migraine-related dizziness or vertigo (benign paroxysmal vertigo of childhood (BPVC), vestibular migraine (VM)), followed by somatoform disorders and head trauma.
- Vertigo or dizziness is extremely common in elderly patients (prevalence rates as high as 33%), with benign paroxysmal positional vertigo (BPPV) being the most common cause of recurrent vertigo.
- In cases with prolonged dizziness, dangerous conditions such as vertebrobasilar stroke or myocardial infarction must be excluded.
- The diagnostic approach to dizziness or vertigo in the geriatric population should include an assessment of current medications, possible triggers, concomitant illnesses, and a general medical examination.

11.1 Falls—obvious, symptomatic, or unexplained?

Here we discuss cases in which sudden, unexplained falls constitute the leading symptom—unexplained, that is, when the cause of the fall is not apparent at first sight. Falls (including those related to syncope or seizure) occur very frequently and make up to 9% of all emergency department (ED) visits. The differential diagnosis of falls is broad; however, only a minority of them are unexplained. In most cases, falls are either secondary to obvious environmental causes (e.g. tripping over obstacles) or are symptomatic, e.g. following transient loss of consciousness (TLOC) or severe vertigo.

11.1.1 Falls—a diagnostic approach

History taking and bedside clinical examination should focus on identifying the most frequent and most dangerous underlying causes of falls (see Table 11.1). Asking about environmental factors (obstacles, slippery ground), pre-existing (movement) disorders, prodromal symptoms, and specific triggers (laughter, head turns, positional changes) may provide valuable information. Patients may report lateropulsion, being pushed or thrown to the ground, or room tilts.

Traditionally, sudden falls without TLOC have been called 'drop attacks'. The term 'drop attack' is variably used for MD, atonic epileptic seizures, and unexplained falls. Some authors apply it to falls in rare subgroups of patients only (falls without TLOC in middle-aged women), whereas others include any fall associated with or without TLOC. Neurotologists often restrict 'drop attacks' to falls resulting from vestibular disorders. Because of these ambiguities it has been suggested that 'drop attacks' should be referred to simply as **sudden falls** with or without TLOC and that 'drop attacks' of apparent vestibular origin should be categorized as either balance-related falls or balance-related near falls (Tarnutzer and Newman-Toker 2013).

11.1.2 Falls related to cardiovascular disorders

Cardiovascular causes of sudden and unexplained falls include cardiac arrhythmias and carotid sinus hypersensitivity. Whether these disorders can lead to sudden falls without TLOC is less certain. However, since TLOC is not always obvious, these disorders may clinically present as unexplained falls.

Contrary to general belief, cardiovascular entities (myocardial infarction, orthostatic hypotension or syncope due to arrhythmia) may often cause vertigo (Newman-Toker *et al* 2008) either in isolation or followed by a fall. Therefore, examination of falls, even

Table 11.1 Differential diagnosis of apparently unexplained falls (modified after Tarnutzer and Newman-Toker 2013)	
Benign or Less Urgent	Dangerous or More Urgent
• Cerebrovascular • Subclavian steal syndrome • Rotational vertebral artery syndrome (RVAS) • Other structural/functional • Chiari malformation, type I • Basilar migraine • Hyperventilation syndrome • Osychogenic pseudo-syncope or non-epileptic seizures • Simple partial seizures • MD (Tumarkin otolithic crisis) • Motor tone disorders (cataplexy, hyperekplexia) • Neurodegenerative postural disorders (e.g. PD, progressive supranuclear palsy, multiple systems atrophy (MSA)) • Psychogenic gait disorders/falls • Cryptogenic falls	• Cerebrovascular • Vertebrobasilar transient ischaemic attack (TIA) • Thalamic ischaemia leading to pusher syndrome or thalamic astasia • Carotid artery occlusion • Subarachnoid haemorrhage • Other structural/functional • Obstructive hydrocephalus • Metabolic (e.g. hypoxia, hypoglycaemia) • Neuroendocrine neoplasm • Acute dystonic reactions (e.g. neuroleptic-induced)

if preceded explicitly by vertigo, should always include an electrocardiogram (ECG) and eventually long term (24 hours or longer) ECG-monitoring.

Carotid artery occlusion and vertebrobasilar TIA are important cerebrovascular causes of unexplained falls. Although either condition may result in loss of consciousness, both tend to cause sudden falls with consciousness preserved. Lesions (most often ischaemic) along the central graviceptive pathways (forwarding signals about the direction of gravity from the vestibular nuclei to the brainstem, thalamus, and cortex) may result in partial or complete ocular tilt reaction, dizziness or vertigo, and ipsiversive or contraversive falls. In Wallenberg syndrome (lateral medullary stroke), lateropulsion towards the side of the lesion may lead to falls in the absence of motor weakness but is typically accompanied by dizziness and other focal brainstem signs (see Chapter 9).

Transient tilts (lasting seconds to hours) of the visual scene—typically by 90 or 180 degrees—in either the roll or pitch plane are referred to as **room-tilt** illusions (see Figure 11.1) and are attributed to a mismatch between visual and vestibular three-dimensional coordinate maps, most frequently observed in brainstem or cortical (ischaemic) lesions (Sierra *et al* 2012).

Substantial misperception of body orientation in the roll plane may be observed in posterolateral thalamic (ischaemic) lesions, leading to imbalance and falls, as in patients with pusher syndrome (Karnath 2007) or thalamic astasia (Brandt and Dieterich 1993). Pusher syndrome describes a condition where patients with lateralized sensorimotor loss due to a thalamic lesion actively push themselves away from the unparalyzed side

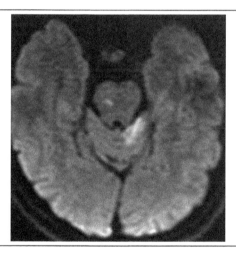

Figure 11.1 Room-tilt illusion secondary to posterior-circulation stroke. This 58-year-old male patient initially presented with a locked-in syndrome due to distal basilar artery occlusion. After local thrombolysis and mechanical thrombectomy, residual complaints on the following day included nausea, dizziness, diplopia, and a 90 degree counter-clockwise room-tilt illusion in the roll plane. Together with the clinical findings (spontaneous left-beating nystagmus) and the magnetic resonance imaging (MRI; demonstrating an acute right paramedian pontine and right cerebellar vermal ischaemia on diffusion-weighted imaging (DWI)), unilateral damage to the ascending graviceptive pathways was proposed. MRI image courtesy of the Department of Neuroradiology, University Hospital Zurich.

using their non-paretic arm or leg. If not prevented, this tendency leads to an unstable laterally-tilted body position and falls. Less frequently, pusher syndrome can also be observed in strokes affecting the insula or the post-central gyrus. In comparison, patients with thalamic astasia present with a tendency to fall backwards or towards the affected side while motor weakness is minor or lacking (Karnath 2007).

A less common cerebrovascular cause for falls is hypoperfusion of the anterior cerebral artery. Subsequent ischaemia in the pre-motor and motor regions controlling the lower extremities can provoke falls without TLOC secondary to leg weakness. Similarly, spinal cord ischaemia (e.g. secondary to aortic dissection) may result in sudden leg weakness and falls. In general, other neurologic symptoms or signs typically accompany sudden falls related to cerebrovascular disorders.

11.1.3 Peripheral vestibular causes

Vestibular diseases may directly cause falls or increase the tendency for falling. The only peripheral vestibular entity which directly causes even dangerous falls, eventually with traumatic injuries such as fractures, is MD. Patients with MD may suffer from 'Tumarkin's otolithic crises': a sudden feeling of being pushed or thrown to the ground or a fall because of a very fast, unexpected vertigo attack or abrupt loss of muscular tone while conscious (probably because of pathologic saccular afferentation). Intratympanal gentamycin therapy successfully stops these attacks together with the classic vertigo spells.

Chronic, unrecognized BPPV, Tullio phenomenon (i.e. sound-induced vertigo and nystagmus related to a third inner-ear window), or bilateral vestibulopathy may add to unsteadiness, thereby increasing the probability of falls.

11.1.4 Symptomatic falls without TLOC

Freezing of gait, narrowing of the base support, and sudden postural failure due to uncompensated shifts in the centre of mass are common causes of falls in movement disorders and (cerebellar or sensory) ataxic syndromes. Sudden, initially unexplained falls can also be secondary to normal pressure hydrocephalus, obstructive hydrocephalus, third ventricle colloid cysts, and tumours of the posterior fossa. Neuroimaging is generally sufficient to identify these structural causes.

Progressively impaired balance and gait and subsequent falls are frequent complaints in extrapyramidal disorders, including both idiopathic (PD) and atypical (MSA, progressive supranuclear palsy (PSP)) Parkinson syndromes and diffuse Lewy body disease.

In PD, risk of falling is about twice as high as in community-based age-matched healthy controls (see Boonstra et al 2008 for a review). Falls in PD are related to loss of postural flexibility ('stiffness'), episodic freezing of gait, lack of compensatory stepping, and proprioceptive disturbances and are typically forward or sideward. Predictors for future falls include prior (near) falls, pathological response on the shoulder pull test (patient requires more than two corrective steps after a single and unexpected shoulder pull backwards), cognitive deficits, high Unified Parkinson's Disease Rating Scale (UPDRS) III score, increased postural sway, and frequent freezing of gate. Falls secondary to syncope (as observed e.g. in MSA-related autonomic dysfunction) are thought to be rare in PD. As impaired balance is an important risk factor for falls in PD patients, physical therapy focusing on intensive balance training should be offered. Exercise and motor training may improve balance-related activities.

Compared to PD, falls are even more frequent and frequent falls (defined as ≥2 falls per year) occur earlier in atypical Parkinson syndromes, reaching 82% in PSP and 59% in MSA (see Chapter 9.6.3). Parkinsonian features, especially postural instability and axial rigidity in combination with mild dementia and supranuclear gaze palsy (initially often limited to slow vertical saccades, later followed by impaired up- and downgaze and eventually by horizontal gaze palsy) are characteristic clinical findings in PSP. Falls tend to be backwards in PSP and may also be related to abnormal otolith-mediated vestibular reflexes. Response to levodopa and other anti-parkinsonian drugs is usually very limited in PSP and MSA.

11.1.5 Psychogenic falls

The spectrum of clinical presentations in psychogenic falls is broad, including complete falls and fall-related (substantial) physical injuries. Young age, very frequent episodes, and falls occurring only in the presence of bystanders are thought to be suggestive for a psychogenic origin. In these patients a history of psychiatric disease, signs of ongoing psychiatric disorders (depression, anxiety), or a history of physical or sexual abuse may further support a psychogenic cause (Reuber et al 2007).

11.1.6 Rare causes of apparently unexplained falls

Rare causes of apparently unexplained falls include **cataplexy** (flaccid falls related to sudden brief bilateral loss of muscle tone due to strong emotions as laughter or surprise), **hyperekplexia** (characterized by exaggerated startle reactions to unexpected stimuli leading to sudden stiff falls), **isolated vestibular epilepsy** (see 9.7), and **cryptogenic drop attacks** (unexplained sudden falls to the knees; in middle-aged women). Consciousness is typically preserved in these conditions. With regards to the differential diagnosis, cataplexy is usually found in patients with narcolepsy. Sudden vestibular falls and atonic seizures are in the differential diagnosis of cataplexy, whereas generalized tonic seizures need to be considered in stiff falls. In patients with suspected cryptogenic drop attacks, triggers or prodromal or postictal symptoms are lacking. The entity of this syndrome remains debated.

11.1.7 Fall precautions

Patients at risk for falls and fall-related injuries should undergo a structured risk assessment including formal gait evaluation. Proposed strategies to prevent falls may include medical treatment (e.g. cataract surgery, implantation of a cardiac pacemaker), elimination of drug-related imbalance, and use of ambulatory assistive devices. Balance training exercises should be considered in all patients with gait imbalance and increased risk for falls and fall-related injuries. Treatment response may be monitored by repetitive formal gait assessment.

11.2 **Dizziness and vertigo in children**

The prevalence of specific disorders leading to dizziness or vertigo changes with age. Some aetiologies are unique to the paediatric population (such as BPVC), and others (such as BPPV, MD) have a much lower rate of occurrence in children than in adults.

The risk of an underlying dangerous condition in patients presenting with vertigo or dizziness to the ED increases significantly with age (<10% at age <25 years vs 25% at age >75 years), including conditions such as cardiac arrhythmia or TIA. Dizziness related to VM or vasovagal syncope peaks in young or middle-aged patients.

Although dizziness, vertigo, and balance disorders are considered less common in the paediatric population (prevalence ranging between 0.4% and 15%) than in adults, they may actually be more common than previously thought (Jahn *et al* 2011). This could be partially explained by a tendency to attribute dizziness or vertigo in children to problems of behaviour or incoordination. Focused patient history and clinical bedside examination are the cornerstones in dizzy children and should include asking for accompanying symptoms (such as headache, hearing problems, focal neurological symptoms), triggers (such as coughing, sneezing, positional changes, stress), and recurrence of symptoms. However, history taking may be limited in young children, if available at all. Furthermore, children are often inexperienced in describing their vestibular complaints as 'dizziness' or 'vertigo'.

In a tertiary vertigo and dizziness centre (paediatric population aged 1–18 years), migraine-related dizziness or vertigo (BPVC or VM) was diagnosed in 36%, somatoform dizziness in 28%, peripheral vestibular lesions in 8%, and vestibular paroxysmia (VP), cerebellar disorders, and orthostatic hypotension in 5% each (Jahn *et al* 2011). Whereas these authors found migraine-related disorders (VM, BPVC) to be the most frequent (> 40%) diagnosis in children aged 7–12 years, the number one diagnosis in adolescents (aged 13–18 years) was somatoform dizziness (reaching > 40%). In a meta-analysis reporting on the most common cases of vertigo or dizziness (McCaslin *et al* 2011), again migraine-related dizziness was diagnosed most frequently (BPVC 19%, VM 17%), followed by head trauma (15%, e.g. secondary to petrous bone fracture, labyrinthine concussion, traumatic BPPV, and perilymph fistula (PLF)), and viral (inner ear) infections (14%). If the neurotological evaluation in the dizzy child remains negative, the clinician must widen the spectrum of differential diagnoses, including disorders such as cardiac arrhythmia, structural heart disorders, drug-related dizziness, anaemia due to occult haemorrhage, and vasovagal syncope.

11.2.1 BPVC

Between the ages of two to six, BPVC is considered the most common cause of episodic vertigo. It usually starts between ages two to four and spontaneous remission by ages five to six is the rule. BPVC belongs to the 'periodic syndromes of childhood that are precursors to migraine'. Short, sudden, and reversible spells of vertigo (lasting seconds to minutes and rarely hours, often occurring in clusters) are characteristic and may be accompanied by anxiety and fear, inability to stand without support, and nausea. In the acute phase, ataxia and spontaneous nystagmus may be observed. Potential triggers include stress, concurrent infections, and motion stimuli. Audio-vestibular work-up in these children rarely shows abnormalities. However, subtle ocular motor signs (such as slightly saccadic smooth pursuit) may be noticed in the interval. Children with BPVC have an increased risk of developing migraine headaches (transformation rate 21–86%) and VM and commonly have a positive family history for migraine (36%) and motion sickness (> 80%). The differential diagnosis of BPVC includes inborn metabolic disorders such as mitochondriopathies and channelopathies (such as episodic ataxia type 2

(EA2)), BPPV, and (less commonly) vestibular neuritis (VN), epileptic vertigo, MD, and posterior fossa tumours. With the spells being short and outcome favourable, most cases will not require specific treatment.

11.2.2 VM

The prevalence of migraine headaches increases dramatically in adolescence: whereas it ranges between 1.2% and 3.2% before age seven, it reaches 8–23% at age 15. About 20% of these children also suffer from vertigo or dizziness, and migraine-related episodic dizziness or vertigo may account for 20–36% of all paediatric cases. Vertigo or dizziness in VM may last a few minutes to several hours and may be accompanied or followed by headaches (although less frequently throbbing and lateralized as in adult migraine patients), photophobia, and phonophobia. However, dizziness or vertigo may present in isolation also (more frequently observed in children aged < 10 years). Lacking migraine treatment guidelines for children, physicians usually adhere to treatment recommendations for adult migraine patients (see Chapter 9).

11.2.3 Motion sickness

Children aged four to ten are the most susceptible to motion sickness. Apparently, persons with an individually increased susceptibility have a tendency to develop migraine in later life. A sensory mismatch between incongruent visual and vestibular input was proposed to explain motion sickness. Treatment options include avoiding situations with conflicting visual and vestibular input, enforcing visual control, and, if required, vestibular suppressants.

11.2.4 Somatoform dizziness in adolescents

In a population-based study of children aged 1–15, a prevalence of 8% for somatoform dizziness was found. In specialized dizzy clinics, somatoform dizziness is diagnosed in 8–25% of cases. It is more frequently observed in adolescents (reaching up to 40% of cases between ages 13 to 17) and may be noted in the context of panic attacks or hyperventilation. These patients may complain of episodic or (more frequently) chronic dizziness along with other vague complaints as shortness of breath, palpitations, and fear. On clinical examination, they may show bizarre or exaggerated limb movements on balance testing. Signs of peripheral or central vestibulopathy, however, are lacking, and vestibular testing is normal. Situational triggering by stress (e.g. at school or crowded places) and ongoing difficulties in relationships may be found. Somatoform dizziness often responds favourably to patient (and parent) education and behavioural advice, with psychotherapy and drug treatment reserved for severe cases.

11.3 **Dizziness and vertigo in the elderly**

The frequency of dizziness and vertigo increases with age and puts the elderly at higher risk of falls and fall-related injuries. Community and primary-care based estimates suggest that 25–33% of adults over 65 have experienced some sort of dizziness, with a one-year prevalence for dizziness of 8–20% in community-dwelling adults at 60 years or older (Barin and Dodson 2011).

Whereas functional decline in the SCCs and the otolith organs does occur with age (Agrawal *et al* 2012), it is still unclear to what extent normal aging of the vestibular system contributes to the increased rates of dizziness and vertigo in the geriatric population in addition to pathological conditions and environmental and lifestyle factors (such as drug-related side effects and polypharmacy).

When evaluating the elderly dizzy patient (Kerber 2010), the high frequency (>80%) of concomitant chronic disorders (such as hypertension, arthritis, and heart disease) that may contribute to or primarily cause dizziness complicates the diagnostic approach. First priority should be to identify dangerous, potentially life-threatening disorders (such as vertebrobasilar stroke, cardiac arrhythmia, and myocardial infarction) and distinguish them from more benign, self-limiting disorders, such as BPPV or orthostatic hypotension. When taking the patient's history (see Chapter 4), assessing current medications, vascular risk factors, and concomitant illnesses is important. The main causes of dizziness in the elderly are: drug-induced dizziness, chronic BPPV, orthostatic hypotension, neurologic diseases due to vascular causes, Parkinson's syndrome, sensory polyneuropathy, and hydrocephalus. The largest fraction (about 50%) of elderly dizzy patients suffers from internal medicine-related disorders. Amongst the peripheral vestibular disorders, BPPV is by far the most common cause in the geriatric population (making up to 40% of all cases above age 70).

References and Further Reading

Agrawal Y., Zuniga M. G., Davalos-Bichara M. *et al.* (2012) Decline in semicircular canal and otolith function with age. *Otol Neurotol.* **33**, 832–9.

Barin K. and Dodson E. E. (2011) Dizziness in the elderly. *Otolaryngol Clin North Am.* **44**, 437–54.

Boonstra T. A., van der Kooij H., Munneke M. *et al.* (2008) Gait disorders and balance disturbances in Parkinson's disease: clinical update and pathophysiology. *Curr Opin Neurol.* **21**, 461–71.

Brandt T. and Dieterich M. (1993) Vestibular falls. *J Vestib Res.* **3**, 3–14.

Jahn K., Langhagen T., Schroeder A. S. *et al.* (2011) Vertigo and dizziness in childhood—update on diagnosis and treatment. *Neuropediatrics.* **42**, 129–34.

Karnath H. O. (2007) Pusher syndrome—a frequent but little-known disturbance of body orientation perception. *J Neurol.* **254**, 415–24.

Kerber K. A. (2010) Dizziness in older people. In: Eggers S. D Z., Zee D. S. (eds). Vertigo and Imbalance: Clinical Neurophysiology of the Vestibular System. Handbook of Clinical Neurophysiology, Vol. 9. Elsevier B.V. pp 491-501.

McCaslin D. L., Jacobson G. P., Gruenwald J. M. (2011) The predominant forms of vertigo in children and their associated findings on balance function testing. *Otolaryngol Clin North Am.* **44**, 291–307.

Newman-Toker D. E., Dy F. J., Stanton V. A. *et al.* (2008) How often is dizziness from primary cardiovascular disease true vertigo? A systematic review. *Gen Intern Med.* **23**, 2087–94.

Reuber M., Howlett S., Khan A. *et al.* (2007) Non-epileptic seizures and other functional neurological symptoms: predisposing, precipitating, and perpetuating factors. *Psychosomatics.* **48**, 230–8.

Sierra-Hidalgo F., de Pablo-Fernández E., Herrero-San Martín A. *et al.* (2012) Clinical and imaging features of the room tilt illusion. *J Neurol.* **259**, 2555–64.

Tarnutzer A. A. and Newman-Toker D. E. (2013) Fits, faints, funny turns, and falls in the differential diagnosis of the dizzy patient. In: Bronstein A. (ed). Vertigo and Imbalance. Oxford Textbook in Clinical Neurology. Oxford University Press, UK. pp 305–30.

Chapter 12

Controversial issues

Key points

- Although arterial loops touching or even distorting the cochleovestibular nerve are frequently seen radiologically, it is questionable as to whether they may cause vertigo attacks.
- Arthritic cervical spine disease is common in the elderly; however, it is disputed as to whether it causes 'cervical' vertigo.
- It is unlikely that hearing loss and vertigo can be caused by rupture of labyrinthine windows (such as the round window) without any clear traumatic precipitating physical event.
- There is a large group of patients with slight chronic postural and/or positional dizziness but with normal vestibular tests. This dizziness may be caused by conditioned/phobic subjective vertigo and/or chronic atypical otoconia displacement.

12.1 Introduction

In neurotology, there are several controversial entities which, being infrequent and lacking well-defined characteristics, remain mysterious even today. These entities arise from the group of unsolved cases with vertigo and dizziness which, in spite of any effort, every specialist encounters in his or her practice. With the advent of new examination methods and the application of new principles (such as the mobile third window syndrome, inferior neuritis, or vestibular migraine (VM)), the percentage of these unsolved cases has decreased. However, there remain a certain number of undiagnosed dizzy patients—usually presenting with slight, chronic dizziness or very short attacks. In both cases, at the time of investigation, no overt vestibular pathology may be found. With careful evaluation, it is usually possible to find some minor alterations, such as an arterial loop in the inner auditory meatus or pathologies of the cervical spine. The strong wish to help on the doctors' side and the chronic, unpleasant, often positional or postural complaints of the patients, which make them feel ill but do not cause abnormal examination results, may combine into theories. Are there perhaps vascular loops in the inner auditory meatus compressing the vestibular nerve and hence causing paroxysmal vertigo attacks? Might pathologic alterations of the cervical spine cause vertigo? Is it possible that spontaneous rupture of the round window membrane causes vertigo and sudden hearing loss? What is behind chronic positional dizziness? Is it a manifestation of migraine? Or, rather, is it purely phobic? Is it caused by dislodged otoconia?

In this section we briefly discuss these questions (without intending to answer them definitively).

12.2 **Vestibular paroxysmia (VP)**

It appears to be a fairly accepted hypothesis that seemingly idiopathic paroxysmal activity of sensory and motor cranial nerves, such as trigeminal neuralgia, hemifacial spasm, and glossopharyngeal neuralgia, may sometimes be caused by vascular compression. In these cases, usually medical therapy with oral anticonvulsants is recommended first.

Sometimes the complaints are resistant and intractable; then operative microvascular decompression using the posterior fossa approach may be offered. Although widely practiced, this entity and its therapeutic procedures may not be considered as unanimously accepted (for an excellent critical review about decompression operations see Monstad 2007). It provoked even more skepticism when the hypothesis of vascular compression was extended to the cochleovestibular nerve (for a review see Yap et al 2008). In 1984, Jannetta et al coined the term 'disabling positional vertigo', consisting of short, repeated, paroxysmal attacks of vertigo lasting seconds to minutes, which can sometimes be provoked by particular head positions. Since these symptoms characterize several entities with dizziness and vertigo (from short attacks of Menière's disease (MD) to atypical benign paroxysmal positional vertigo (BPPV)) and because it has not been possible to define reliable diagnostic criteria, the theory that vascular loops may compress the vestibular nerve and cause short spontaneous or positional vertigo attacks remains controversial. It was one of the greatest peers of neurotology ever, Harold Schuknecht from Harvard University, who, on the basis of his pathological observations, called it a myth that 'vascular loops should be considered as a possible cause for otherwise unexplained otologic symptoms' (Schuknecht 1992). Apparently, on high-resolution magnetic resonance imaging (MRI), loops of the anterior inferior cerebellar artery (AICA) are very frequently seen in contact with the cochleovestibular nerve, even in healthy, asymptomatic persons (e.g. 20% of normals). In the literature, the apparent effectivity of carbamazepine in cases with short, paroxysmal vertigo spells has been cited in favour of the theory. However, controlled, systematic studies are missing. Spontaneous improvement is always possible even without the pathogenic role of arterial compression, and eventually the role of other diagnostic entities (such as BPPV) may be postulated.

12.3 **Cervical vertigo**

Neck afferents deliver inputs to the vestibular system. In animal studies, it was possible to elicit a cervico-ocular reflex originating from receptors in ligaments and capsules of articulations. The reflex, however, has a low gain (0.1) (for a review see Baloh and Kerber 2011), and its role in pathological processes has not been elucidated yet (for a balanced review see Brandt and Bronstein 2001). There is evidence that this reflex helps to stabilize gaze following vestibular damage as its gain increases after bilateral loss of vestibular function. As SCC afferents and neck afferents converge on the secondary neurons of the vestibular nuclei in the brainstem, vibration of neck muscles induces changes in body movements and visual orientation. Dysfunction of these afferents therefore might cause 'cervical vertigo'. However, it is uncertain if such a purely cervical 'vertigo' or dizziness exists at all.

There are several pathological entities with vertigo on head turning, such as the rotational vertebral artery syndrome (RVAS; see Section 9.3.5), vertebral artery dissection (VAD; see Section 9.3.1) and Arnold-Chiari malformation with neck pain (see Section 9.6.1.5). In other cases, light, short dizzy spells (lasting seconds) and cervical pain coexist, such as in Lyme disease. It is, however, questionable as to whether isolated neck pathology (degenerative or rheumatic) may cause vertigo or dizziness. First, there seems to be no diagnostic test as an unambiguous criterion. Second, although arthritic changes of the cervical spine are frequent with increasing age, it is difficult to correlate them to vertigo complaints. Third, usually there is some other possible explanation, such as in post-traumatic cervical vertigo, when after a whiplash injury, complaints may usually be explained by accompanying slight traumatic brainstem injuries or by post-traumatic BPPV due to dislodged otoconia.

12.4 **Spontaneous perilymphatic fistula**

Hearing loss and dizziness occur when perilymph oozes out of the vestibulum into the middle ear, either through one of the physiological windows of the inner ear (the oval window with the stapes in it, and the round window) or through a third traumatic opening. Traumatic perilymph fistula (PLF), due to fracture of the stapes in the oval window (through an accident or ear operation) or penetrating injury around the round window, is a relatively well-defined entity. Sometimes even air bubbles can be identified in the cochlea or the vestibulum on high-resolution computed tomography (CT) images of the temporal bone (pneumolabyrinth). Barotraumas (such as with diving accidents) may apparently also cause inner ear injuries. Antonelli et al (1993) found a haemorrhage around Reissner's membrane and the round window membrane and rupture of the utricle and saccule. However, these cases stemmed from barotraumas, when the scuba diver actually died in the diving accident. Whereas **middle ear** dysfunction due to barotrauma caused by insufficient pressurization is common in divers or during flights in high altitude, it seems that isolated **inner ear** barotraumas causing hearing loss and vertigo may be rare after all.

Even more uncertainties arise when authors try to explain seemingly idiopathic sudden hearing loss and accompanying dizziness with spontaneous PLF (for a review see Merchant et al 2008).

Idiopathic sudden hearing loss (ISHL) has resisted efforts in the last decades to be characterized and remains a mysterious and controversial entity. Because it improves spontaneously in possibly 40–70% of cases and because it lacks proven pathogenic mechanisms, it is difficult to assess therapeutic effects. Earlier it was postulated that ISHL might perhaps sometimes occur due to the sudden rupture of the round window membrane. In these cases (usually with sudden profound hearing loss), operative treatment was attempted (by closure of the round window membrane). However, even when it occurred during some physical activity with exertion (such as weight lifting, sneezing), and therefore a causal connection could be assumed between the hearing loss and sudden intracranial pressure increase, it was difficult to document perilymph leaking. Perilymph has a small volume (under 0.1 ml), and an eventual leak is hard to visualize even when attempts are made to augment it by intrathecally administered fluorescein (Gehrking et al 2002).

As Merchant et al (2008) cautiously put it: 'There are several lines of argument to indicate that a break of labyrinthine membranes is not a common cause of ISHL, including clinical, experimental and histopathologic lines of evidence.' They also state that 'middle ear exploration, which used to be commonly performed in patients with ISHL for presumed oval or round window ruptures, has been largely given up in the USA, in part because of negative results.' Apparently, in cases without any clear traumatic precipitating physical event which might have led to the hearing loss, other mechanisms have to be assumed. The authors suggest the 'stress response' theory. According to this hypothesis, abnormal stimulation of cellular stress pathways within the cochlea could cause ISHL, starting with pathological activation of transcription factors (i.e. nuclear factor-κB), which in turn could be elicited, for instance, by a systemic viral illness producing enhanced levels of cytokines or reactive oxygen species (Merchant et al 2008).

12.5 **Chronic postural/positional dizziness**

There is a rather large group of patients who chronically experience dizziness even though all vestibular tests are practically normal. In this group, symptoms are occasionally persistent and sometimes may wax and wane spontaneously. When present, fluctuating episodes of unsteadiness last seconds to minutes or momentary perceptions of illusory body motions, most severely when walking or standing, may occur. Sometimes, unsteadiness may be accentuated by situations when immediate visual clues are missing (i.e., in open spaces, on bridges). In the nineties of the last century, Brandt et al (1994) attributed these symptoms to a 'transient uncoupling of efference and efference copy, leading to a mismatch between anticipated and actual motion' in persons with an obsessive-compulsive personality, anxiety, and vegetative disturbance (for a review see Brandt 1996). They suggested a therapy that consisted of relieving the patients of their fear of organic disease in consultative sessions by explaining to them the hypothetical mechanism. They coined the term 'phobic postural vertigo' for this condition.

Based on these results, later Staab and Ruckestein (2007) conducted their own studies and described the so-called 'chronic subjective dizziness' (CSD), a very similar entity, consisting of persistent non-vertiginous dizziness lasting three months or more, hypersensitivity to motion stimuli, including a patient's own movement and motion of objects in the visual surrounds, and difficulty with precision visual tasks such as reading or using a computer (for a review see Staab 2012). The authors found a high prevalence of psychiatric disorders (93%) among patients with CSD, which contributed to their symptoms, and they suggested serotonin reuptake inhibitors as a potential treatment.

In the groups, which were created in attempts to differentiate dizziness syndromes that could not be explained by known neurotologic disorders, complaints were aggravated by **posture**. Body posture is of course closely associated with head position and head movements. There have been made efforts to characterize subjective dizziness elicited by **positional** stimuli. The definition of BPPV requires vertical-torsional positional nystagmus evoked by the Dix-Hallpike manoeuvre or predominantly horizontal positional nystagmus after rolling the head sideways from the supine position. However, neurotologists regularly see patients with typical complaints of BPPV but without positioning nystagmus. In 2012, Büki et al noted that such patients, although having typical BPPV symptoms (short vertigo when bending forward, lying down, sitting up or turning over in bed) rarely complain of vertigo (and do not have nystagmus) in the Dix-Hallpike position, but do experience short vertigo spells during the act of sitting up and for a short time immediately afterwards. They sometimes even have abnormal antero- and retropulsion and trunk oscillations during sitting up. This sitting-up vertigo was typically unilateral; that is, it predominantly occurred during sitting up from the right or left Dix-Hallpike position, carried out either in the left anterior right posterior (LARP) or in the right anterior left posterior (RALP) plane. This, according to the authors, made other mechanisms, such as orthostatic dysregulation, changes in intracranial pressure, or increased motion sensitivity, improbable. The authors suggested that this so-called 'type 2 BPPV' might be elicited by otoconial debris in the short arm of the posterior canal. In classical BPPV, otoconia fall off the utricular macula, usually when the patient is in a supine position. During the night, when the utricular macula is upside down, there is a greater probability of otoconial displacement. This is possibly why classical canalolithiasis frequently starts in the morning, when the patient sits up for the first time. However, during the day there may also be smaller particles which dislodge. If this occurs in an upright posture, the otoconia necessarily roll along the utricle and gravitate toward the most inferior part of the vestibule, which is the ampulla of the posterior canal (for a three-dimensional anatomical reconstruction, see the upper panel of Figure 6.11). In the ampulla, the debris fall onto the cupula, making it chronically sensitive to linear accelerations. During examination in the head-hanging position, no nystagmus ensues, but the chronically sensitized cupula acts paradoxically during sitting up. Also, when sitting up, the debris falling back onto the cupula may cause trunk sway for a second.

For therapy, the authors recommended repetitive sit-ups from the Dix-Hallpike positions. The head-hanging position during this manoeuvre is supposed to liberate the short arm of the posterior canal from canaliths. Because of the normally low endolymphatic calcium concentration, movements of the debris should speed up their dissolution. Interestingly, in many cases strong vegetative symptoms (sweating, nausea and even retching) emerge at the beginning of the training, which is certainly out of proportion considering the subtlety of the manoeuvres. If the patients continue to apply this liberation manoeuvre, these unpleasant symptoms soon disappear. Sometimes, even prophylactic antivertiginous therapy may be needed to be given for a few days before starting the liberation manoeuvres.

Possibly there is some overlapping between phobic postural vertigo, subjective, chronic dizziness, and subliminal, chronic (type 2) BPPV. The size of displaced, pathologic debris hypothetically shows a continuous distribution from very small to bigger particles, and there may be a certain intermediate mass which is big enough to cause subjective complaints but too small to elicit overt symptoms and signs such as nystagmus.

It will be difficult to decide on this issue in the future. By suffering from chronic positional symptoms, people may be sensitized/conditioned against specific head movements and show avoiding behaviour. Slight, repetitive positional symptoms may

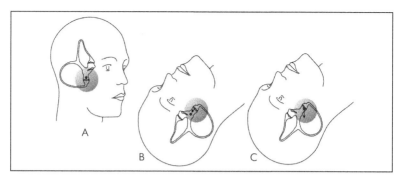

Figure 12.1 The hypothetical mechanism of type 2 BPPV. A. In an upright position, the debris is deposited on the cupula of the posterior canal. B. In type 2 BPPV without downbeat positional nystagmus, the debris falls down off the cupula. C. If the debris adheres to the cupula, peripheral positional downbeat nystagmus may develop (see also Figure 6.5).

generalize into postural avoidance. It is also possible that the repetitive sit-ups do not act through the proposed hypothetical short arm liberation, but simply by habituation/desensitization. Interestingly, when patients with CSD carry out physical rehabilitation therapy, it has to be gentle at the beginning; otherwise it exacerbates complaints (Staab 2012). This may correspond to the out-of-proportion vegetative symptoms in type 2 BPPV.

In a recent paper, Cambi et al (2013) studied peripheral positional downbeat nystagmus elicited by Dix-Hallpike or straight head-hanging position. Apparently, this kind of benign and spontaneously improving nystagmus may be more frequent than previously thought and may not exclusively be caused by anterior canal cupulo-canalolithiasis. As an explanation, the authors evoke the hypothesis of the type 2 BPPV, the short arm canalolithiasis. Indeed, positional, peripheral downbeat nystagmus may be a special case of type 2 BPPV, that of a short arm **cupulo**lithiasis, when debris attached to the cupula may pull it in the direction of the utriculus in the head-hanging position as also discussed in Chapter 6 (Figure 12.1).

A particularly impressive argument in favour of this hypothesis was that the authors noticed a high association (30%) of downbeat nystagmus to previous or subsequent ipsilateral posterior canalolithiasis. This showed that the peripheral downbeat nystagmus had something to do with freely moving particles in the utriculus. Interestingly, in 1962, in his first original paper about BPPV, Schuknecht described the same putative mechanism as a possible cause (see also Baloh 2001), because in the pathological specimens he saw deposits on the utricular side of the cupula (Figure 12.2). Of course, it was impossible to explain the nystagmus in **canalo**lithiasis by this theory, as discussed by Baloh (2001). However, with hindsight, his pathological observations were correct, and today, thanks to the results of otoconia research, three-dimensional labyrinth reconstructions and three-dimensional vector-nystagmography, a conclusive picture emerges that will contribute to the development of effective therapy for BPPV.

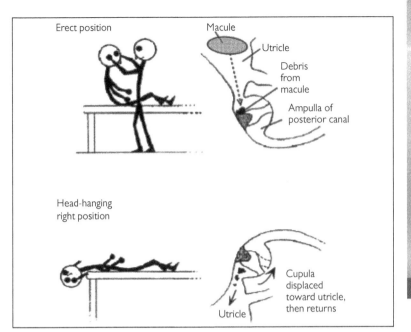

Figure 12.2 Schuknecht's hypothesis concerning BPPV as cited by Baloh (2001), showing Schuknecht's original presentation from 1961. Reprinted from Baloh R. W. (2001). © 2001, with permission from Wolters Kluwer Health.

References and Further Reading

Agarwal K., Bronstein A. M., Faldon M. E. et al. (2012) Visual dependence and BPPV. J Neurol. **259**, 1117–24.

Antonelli P. J., Parell G. J., Becker G. D. et al. (1993) Temporal bone pathology in scuba diving deaths. Otolaryngol Head Neck Surg. **109**, 514–21.

Baloh R. W. (2001) Harold Schuknecht and pathology of the ear. Otol Neurotol. **22**, 113–22.

Baloh R. W. and Kerber K. A. (2011) Clinical Neurophysiology of the vestibular system, 4th edn. Oxford University Press.

Brandt T. (1996) Phobic postural vertigo. Neurology. **46**, 1515–9.

Brandt T. and Bronstein A. M. (2001) Cervical vertigo. J Neurol Neurosurg Psychiatry. **71**, 8–12.

Brandt T., Huppert D., Dieterich M. (1994) Phobic postural vertigo: a first follow-up. J Neurol. **241**, 191–5.

Büki B., Simon L., Garab S. et al. (2012) Sitting-up vertigo and trunk retropulsion in patients with benign positional vertigo but without positional nystagmus. J Neurol Neurosurg Psychiatry. **82**, 98–104.

Cambi J., Astore S., Mandalà M. et al. (2013) Natural course of positional down-beating nystagmus of peripheral origin. J Neurol [Epub ahead of print].

Gehrking E., Wisst F., Remmert S. *et al.* (2002) Intraoperative assessment of perilymphatic fistulas with intrathecal administration of fluorescein. *Laryngoscope.* **112**, 1614–8.

Jannetta P. J., Møller M. B., Møller A. R. (1984) Disabling positional vertigo. *N Engl J Med.* **310**, 1700–5.

Merchant S. N., Durand M. L., Adams J. C. (2008) Sudden deafness: is it viral? *ORL J Otorhinolaryngol Relat Spec.* **70**, 52–60.

Monstad P. (2007) Microvascular decompression as a treatment for cranial nerve hyperactive dysfunction—a critical view. *Acta Neurol Scand Suppl.* **187**, 30–3.

Schuknecht H. F. (1962) Positional vertigo: clinical and experimental observations. *Trans Am Acad Ophthalmol Otol.* **66**, 319–31.

Schuknecht H. F. (1992) Myths in neurotology. *Am J Otol.* **13**, 124–6.

Staab J. P. (2012) Chronic subjective dizziness. *Continuum.* **18**, 1118–41.

Staab J. P. and Ruckenstein M. J. (2007) Expanding the differential diagnosis of dizziness. *Arch Otolaryngol Head Neck Surg.* **133**, 170–6.

Yap L., Pothula V. B., Lesser T. (2008) Microvascular decompression of cochleovestibular nerve. *Eur Arch Otorhinolaryngol.* **265**, 861–9.

Index